AGING YOUR BEST
UNTIL YOU STOP

What to expect
and what to do about it

DANNY KUHN

ISBN: 978-1-7372953-4-1

$16.95 USD

Copyright © 2024 Danny Kuhn

Favoritetrainers.com Books

Myrtle Beach, South Carolina USA

Cover image: Skull of a Skeleton with Burning Cigarette by
Vincent van Gogh, 1886 PUBLIC DOMAIN

COVER DESIGN BY SETH ELLISON

DEDICATION

This book is dedicated to the memory of W. Mark Deskins, who died suddenly and unexpectedly at the age of 64 during its writing. From growing up in the coalfields of West Virginia, he became an accomplished engineer and a senior manager for the Department of the Navy. All along the way, he was a worthy role model and true friend to many, including me. "Most of the time, I choose to look forward instead of back" he said.

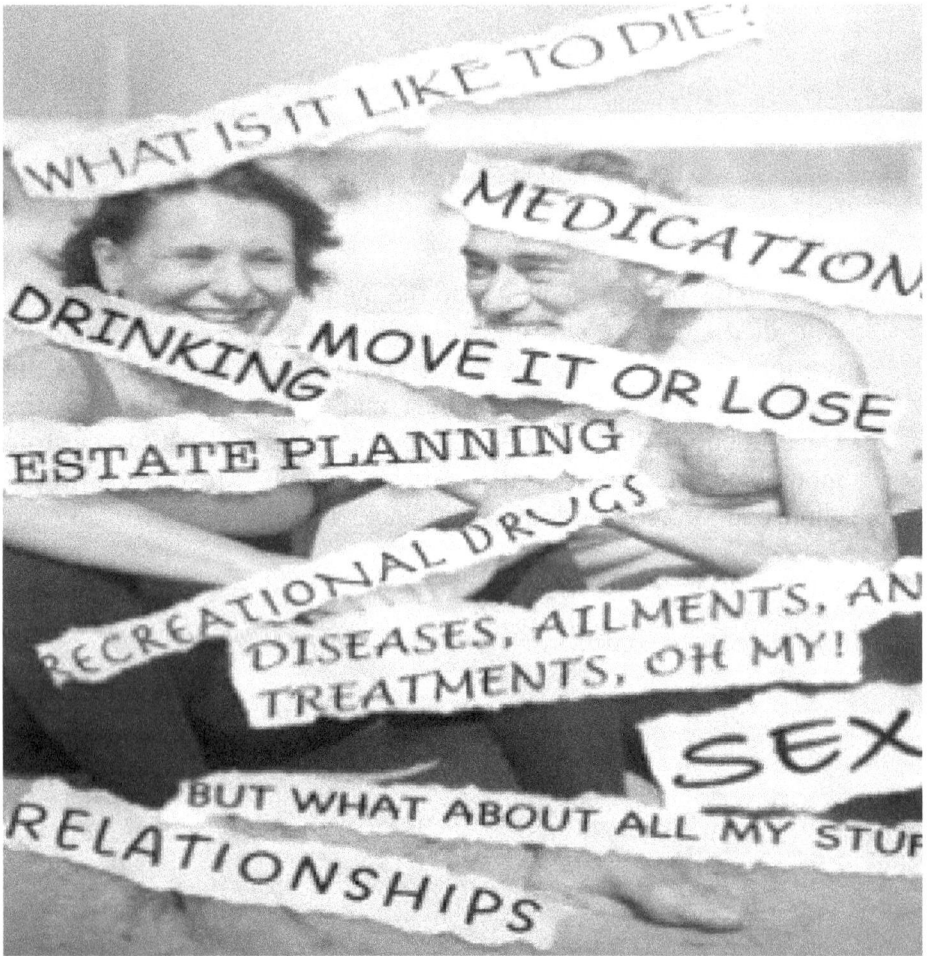

CONTENTS

PROLOGUE: YOU KNOW HOW THIS ENDS

You're going to die, and it will probably be sooner than it has been. But there are things you can do to make the time you have left better.

Don't like the aging process? No worries. It will be over for you relatively soon, in the big scheme of things. That's not optional. Know what to expect and how to plan and react.

So many things began slowly changing for me in my 60s, so I did what I always do. I read and researched. Outside of informative but dry clinical works by doctors and academics, though, most of the popular books I found on aging were of the "Find Your Passion! Share Your Wisdom! Now's Your Time! BEST SEX EVER!" variety.

Yeah, right. You and I obviously weren't born yesterday. What I really need is someone to give me honest information, best-practice options, and fact-based explanation without pushing the pollyannaish, feelgood, sunny scenario "take those aging, shriveled, desiccated lemons life gave you and you forgot about in the back of your refrigerator and make refreshing, reinvigorating LEMONADE and maybe even LEMONDROP COCKTAILS for a romantic evening!" false narrative.

Don't get me wrong. It's not all doom and gloom. Addressing and anticipating those not-so-pleasant things that may (and most likely will) happen and preparing for them mentally, physically, financially, spiritually, and every other -ally can improve not only your quality of life, but that of your loved ones.

I'm not a doctor, nor a financial planner, nor a psychologist, nor a sex therapist nor a gerontologist, but I have spent most of my life researching trustworthy sources and communicating information to others in a useable *and readable* format. I am also willing to tell you things about aging you probably already know and fear and for that reason choose to ignore. You need to be reminded, straight up. I'm that friend-from-childhood you are talking with around the fire pit after a few drinks, the one who loves you like a sibling but no longer feels any need to tiptoe around in our conversations: sometimes you love him for it; other times, you temporarily despise him as a preachy buttinsky. But you know what he's saying is valid.

What do either of us have to lose? Read the first two sentences of this introduction again. Sometimes we become a little forgetful as we age, so I'll remind you along the way.

This material is neither erotic nor particularly graphic, but please note it is honest and specific, about sex and death and everything in between. I occasionally find and share some humor and personal experiences even while addressing those very personal, yet universal, topics. Be advised.

1 PUT SEX BACK ON THE TABLE

You're going to die, and it will probably be sooner than it has been. But there are things you can do to make the time you have left better.

No, that's not what I mean by *on the table*, and you know it. Unless, of course, it's what you want. It's your table and none of my business.

Why did you begin with sex? an early reviewer of this book asked me. *Gee. I thought we all did,* I replied. Besides, a lot of the rest of the book deals with things more likely to kill you, so let's dwell in that happier place before we must abandon it.

> *"I used to exercise, but I don't anymore. I can't do it the way I could when I was 20; it's more difficult and not as much fun, I don't look as good doing it as I used to, and I don't have a regular partner to do it with now. I know it's good for me and can even help me live longer, but I've lost interest and it's not worth the bother."*

You already see where I am going with this, don't you? It's probably unnecessary, but let's complete the thought process anyway. Substitute "have sex" for "exercise" in the passage:

"I used to have sex, but I don't anymore. I can't do it the way I could when I was 20; it's more difficult and not as much fun, I don't look as good doing it as I used to, and I don't have a regular partner to do it with now. I know it's good for me and can even help me live longer, but I've lost interest and it's not worth the bother."

From a health, happiness, and longevity prospective, the second paragraph makes no more sense than the first. It's just as harmful, just as lazy, just as defeatist, and just as dangerous. Get over it.

Sexual satisfaction is not just for the young. Or the fit. Or the fully abled. Or the attractive in the eyes of popular culture. Or the partnered. Or the genitally fully functioned. Sexual satisfaction is an essential element of human experience, and a basic human right. Not seizing it to whatever degree you can is a waste of a great gift, a rejection of our nature, an invitation to mental and physical infirmity, and may even shorten your life. It is also almost always unnecessary.

Senior sexuality is most often portrayed as comical, an object of derision, or even disgust. It's your job (and mine) to disprove that ignorant, bigoted myth, and as soon as possible. Maybe tonight. Or even better, this afternoon!

BEST SEX EVER!

Uh huh. Sure thing. While television and movies make fun of senior sex to the point that even we older folks feel ashamed to talk about it, some books and articles aimed at seniors in the popular media target false hope to get you to buy something. Sex can (and should) be great at our age, but *best sex ever*? Come on, man. And woman. I mean, that unexpectedly sexy night at a local hotel with your partner after the water line to the refrigerator busted and you had to vacate your house was a real pleasure. Maybe you still make little jokes about it a year later, but do you replay it in your mind the way you do scenes from that weekend in August 1977 when you went to the Peter Frampton concert in Cleveland with your girlfriend or boyfriend while your parents thought you were camping with your cousin? Answer honestly. And if a night in a hotel thanks to a flooded floor made that much difference, maybe you should get a stylish set of numbers and attach them to your bedroom door.

Frankly, be glad we seniors DON'T have the best sex ever. Before you dismiss that as blasphemous or self-hating, hear me out: If, as we continue through life, we remained as driven, as obsessed with sex as we were at 20, I doubt society would be so advanced. We wouldn't have given other things nearly as much thought and energy if sex kept getting better and better and better until it was time for the undertaker to undo the smiles on our faces so mourners wouldn't be tempted to make lewd jokes. We need the added cognitive space to think about when best to take Social Security, whether to rent a convertible Mustang to drive to our 50th reunion, who got grandma's cast iron skillet instead of you (who she really meant to have it!), and other important things. Adjusting our clothing at inopportune times, sleeping with someone's photograph on the pillow beside us, and sneaking out at night to draw hearts on the sidewalk in front of someone's house are all time consuming and could interfere with our weekly Bunco game.

But the grand thing is that it doesn't have to be the *best sex ever* to add pleasure, and maybe even years, to your life, and it's easier than you may think to revive this free benefit even under personal circumstances most would not consider optimal. It's a matter of will, adaptability, and managed expectations. Let's look at what's going on, the medical science behind the benefits, and how we can make it at least *better*.

ARE WE STILL, YOU KNOW, DOING IT?

When I first began researching senior sexuality, it seemed like there is a plethora of scientific information, or maybe three-fourths of a plethora, at least. But then I found most of the articles were really restatements of one big study done as part of the University of Michigan's *Institute for Healthcare Policy and Innovation's National Poll on Healthy Aging*, an ongoing project partially supported by the American Association of Retired Persons. Yes, that's right, friends. We have progressed from *Penthouse*

Forum to the AARP as a source for sex information. Congratulations.

Of the participants in the study (all in the United States) aged 65-80, 72% reported having a romantic partner. Overall, 40% said they are currently sexually active, with a higher percentage (46%) in the younger end of the demographic, falling to only 25% of the 76–to-80-year-olds. Men were 20% more likely to respond they are sexually active than women. Perhaps not surprisingly, the higher the respondents ranked their overall health, the higher their chances of being sexually active. Half of the men described themselves as being extremely or very interested in sex, but only 12% of the women said the same. Nearly three fourths (73%) said they were either extremely, very, or somewhat satisfied with their sex life, with women being more likely to be extremely satisfied than men. (1)

That's quite a bit to digest, and not particularly uplifting, no pun intended. The overall rate of being sexually active is dismal, at least to my thinking.

There were jobs and kids and everything else for all those years, but by the time the kids were gone and we had more time together, we had just kind of gotten out of the habit, I guess. – Female

When it comes to sexual practices, I know you want the lowdown, don't you?

For example, how often? A *New England Journal of Medicine* study (2) polled 3,005 American adults (slightly more woman than men) aged 57 to 85 in 2004. Only eight of the respondents reported being in a same-sex relationship. The study revealed that among people aged 75-85 who were sexually active, 54% reported having sex two or three times per month, and 23% said they do it once or more per week.

You go, gang! But remember, that only reflects those who report being sexually active, not the overall senior population.

How often is one thing, but exactly what, pray tell, are these seniors doing? Those naughty numbers require even more digging, and that's a problem. It seems that specific sex practices among our age group have not been studied as thoroughly as in others. We can find loads of statistics about non-intercourse sexual practices, same sex or group activity, pornography use, etc. among teenagers, for example, but the full scope of similar information about seniors is more difficult to find. The research published in the *New England Journal of Medicine* cited above also found that 52% of men and 25% of women with an intimate partner polled reported masturbating (defined as "stimulating your genitals {sex organs} for sexual pleasure not with a partner) in the previous year, as compared to 55% of men and 23% of women who were not in an intimate relationship. Of the sexually active, 58% of the respondents in the youngest segment of the poll population reported having had oral sex in the past year, as compared with 31% in the oldest group.

And that desire thingy? In the study, just over a third of women rated sex as "not at all important," while only 13% of men said the same.

For those who have a partner but have not had sex within the past three months, the (obviously overlapping, given the numbers) reasons included:

Lack of interest - 19%

Interested, but partner is not - 17%

Religious beliefs - 9%

Lack of opportunity - 2%

Understandably, the natural effects of aging loomed large in respondents' answers, with 61% citing health problems or limitations, and 23% citing their partner's limitations. We will look at all these things more closely.

Dang, that sounded weird.

WHY IT MATTERS: THE BENEFITS OF HAVING SEX

We usually aren't aiming to have babies anymore, unless you're Robert De Niro, whose latest one came along while he was age 79. Yeah, I'm talkin' to you. Good for him, but he gives a good reminder to us guys that you never age out on the importance of contraception. Australian Les Colley (1898-1998) fathered a child (his ninth) at age 92, with a woman he met through a dating agency.

But, yes, whatever your age, it really does matter for both mental and physical health, and the science is unambiguous.

YOUR MIND: We will start with the brain and work our way down, so to speak. The Universities of Oxford and Coventry in England aren't fly-by-night institutions offering online degrees in Jellied Eel Studies, so we can trust their methodology. In 2016, the universities conducted a joint study that linked senior sexual activity with higher cognitive abilities as one ages. It involved participants aged 50-83 using two standard tests: number sequencing relating to the brain's executive functions, and word recall relating to memory. The results were sorted and adjusted as to participants' ages within the group, gender, education level, and other factors that may affect results. The study found continued sexual activity is strongly linked to improved performance in both number sequencing and word recall in the male respondents, and in word recall among the female respondents.

Bob, I couldn't think of the name of that green turnip-like thing that tastes like broccoli at the grocery store this afternoon. You know what we need to do! (smiles slyly)
It's kohlrabi, Miriam. Kohlrabi.

The results were graduated: the more sex, the better the scores. You can see the full results in *The Journals of Gerontology, Series B: Psychological and Social Sciences*, June 22, 2017. (3)

Now let's go down...under. A study of more than 6,000 subjects with a median age of 66 was performed under the auspices of the University of Wollongong, New South Wales, and then repeated two years later, being published in 2018. (4) It showed a strong relationship between sexual activity and memory performance.

So, what's going on? More research needs to be done (where can I sign up?), but the Oxford/Coventry study suggests one connection may be the increased levels of the hormones dopamine and oxytocin that are released during sex. These brain chemicals may play a role in improving the communication between brain regions. Just how it happens is yet to be fully understood, and we still know more about the results than we do about the mechanisms. An Italian study (Sexual Life of 352 Elderly Italians Aged 65-105 Years) reinforces that notion. (5)

Why does even writing the words "Sexual Life" in the same sentence as a reference to 105-year-old Italians remind me of conversations around the bar after a Knights of Columbus meeting? You had to be there.

That's cognition. For emotional health, the connection is even stronger.

"Sexual Activity is Associated with Greater Enjoyment of Life in Older Adults." *No DUH.* In that article (6) the researchers, building on the English Longitudinal Study of Aging that has now been going on for two decades with almost 20,000 participants over that time, used a proven life-enjoyment instrument called the CASP-19 (Control, Autonomy, Self-realization, and Pleasure) inventory to measure life quality among 3,045 men and 3.834 women, with a mean age of around 65. Respondents who reported sexual activity within the past year scored a significantly higher mean in enjoyment of life compared to those who did not.

There is an interesting finding, however, in the scores of men vs. women when it comes to the benefit of different *kinds* of intimate activity. For the men, frequent intercourse (defined as two or more times per month) and frequent non-intercourse intimacy (defined as kissing, petting, or fondling) were both associated with greater enjoyment of life. With women, those non-intercourse activities were as well, but there was no significant association between life enjoyment and frequent actual intercourse vs. other physical intimacy.

Interesting…but surprising? The male/female divide about the importance of cuddling and touch does not, if you haven't noticed, suddenly appear on one's fiftieth birthday. And, as defined in the study, "kissing, petting, or fondling" can include intimate acts that go a long, long way towards full sexual satisfaction. *Looong way. Everything BUT….*

For some, the definition of "having sex" could simply be broader and more inclusive as we progress in life. Get it? I will see your "any physical contact between two persons that involves stimulation of the genitals of either one or both participants" and raise you a "various activities like masturbation, foreplay, kissing, or anything that a person might find arousing." The brain doesn't distinguish between "partnered intercourse dopamine and oxytocin" and "relaxed and alone in my bedroom still thinking about that Peter Frampton concert dopamine and oxytocin" if you get my drift. Hormones be hormones, sisters and brothers. They gonna do what they gonna do.

But the results are clear, and positive. There is a connection between having sex and staying sharp and happy as you age. Because of the hormones it releases, sex in whatever form reduces stress and anxiety. It can boost your mood, both because of brain chemistry and feelings of attachment, purpose, relevance, security, and, especially as we age, even *accomplishment*. It can improve cognitive abilities and help rebuild self-confidence and self-esteem that sometimes suffer in our stage of life.

You've still got it, baby. It might take longer to prime and take more pulls on the cord to start the engine, but you've still got it.

I look at it like this: my husband and I like to eat nice meals. Bad things come from not eating. Of course, bad things can come from eating too much, or the wrong way. We usually enjoy eating together, and like many of the same things. There are also things each of us like but the other doesn't. Now, sometimes there is room for compromise. He no longer picks the cucumber slices out of salads, and I tolerate a thin dollop of guacamole on my nachos. But I'm not eating sardines, period. Likewise, onion soup for him, and that's okay. Some meals are better than others, leisurely with steak and asparagus, but sometimes just a quick grilled cheese. It's all good! We sometimes eat together even if we've had a disagreement, or are a bit tired or distracted, or would rather watch a Hallmark movie or a ball game; we still do it. If either of us is hungry but the other isn't, no one minds if we make a quick sandwich just for ourselves. Heaven forbid, if one of us is without the other someday, that's no reason for whoever's left to never eat again, now is it? (scoffs) You do know I'm really talking about sex, right? -Female

You are wise, Female. The positive effects of sex for your body should be even more obvious than those on your mind. After all, sexual activity is *activity*, something modern humans often have too little of regardless of the type. It may not be the same as going to the gym and walking on the treadmill or riding those uncomfortable stationary bicycles or swimming laps, but it beats the heck out of sitting on the couch and watching Netflix without the chill.

Sex, with a partner or alone, increases your heart rate. This, in turn, can strengthen the heart muscle and help it pump blood more efficiently and lower your blood pressure. The release of endorphins, in addition to enhancing mood as we already noted, can even give temporary relief to chronic pain.

Sex, with a partner or alone, burns calories. A study by the University of Montreal in 2013 (7) concluded that lovemaking burns approximately 3.1 calories per minute for women, and 4.2 calories for men.

Two reactions: 1) Individual results may vary, and the subjects in this study were young couples; and 2) Again, where do I sign up for these studies? But, since these couples were all wired up to monitors during their energy expenditure, maybe I will pass on this one.

Walking on a treadmill will burn, on average, just over ten times more calories per minute, but which minute will you be more likely to remember fondly when you're deciding whether to heed the call to "come into the light?"

Sex, with a partner or alone, may help you sleep better. An important study verifying this "thing we already knew" (8) included 787 participants and suggests the biochemical mechanism: Sex increases the hormones oxytocin and prolactin, and reduces cortisol, the stress response hormone that can cause poor sleep quality and is strongly associated with cardiovascular disease and metabolic disorders. Not sleeping as well as we used to is a common complaint at almost all ages, certainly including seniors, and it can be linked to several maladies, both physical and mental. Cortisol can make you tired and irritable, and even tempted to drink more than you should or take sleep meds that have side effects.

It's about time this study was done. Until 2020, most of our scientific verification of the very intuitive connection between sex and sleep had been conducted on rats, and I suppose the white coats had finally seen enough of male rats rolling over and snoring loudly while their female counterparts looked miffed.

Adequate sleep can also be a factor in the next sex benefit:

Sex, with a partner or alone, can boost your immune system. Our immune system and avoiding infection practically consumed our thinking for almost two years, during the COVID-19 pandemic. Hats off to the researchers who realized that was the perfect time to do an incredibly broad (16,000 participants spread over 33 countries) survey of the connection between sexual activity and contracting the virus. (9) There was a strong correlation between the frequency of one's sexual activity and not becoming infected with COVID-19, as well as milder symptoms among those who did become infected, or, in the words of the study, "As one's sexual activity increases, the immunity status becomes more competent to deal with pathogens."

More than one study, including that by Carl J. Charnetski and Francis X. Brennan in association with Wilkes University in Wilkes-Barre, Pennsylvania, found higher concentrations of salivary immunoglobulin A (IgA) in the saliva of participants who reported having frequent sex. IgA (not to be confused with the grocery store) is an antibody found in the mucous membranes of the lungs, sinuses, stomach and intestines and the fluids those membranes produce. It plays a significant role in protecting us from all sorts of infectious microorganisms.

Sex, with a partner or alone, can help you remain continent. A woman's pelvic floor muscles accomplish incredible tasks, and over the years may, like other muscles, weaken if not exercised and strengthened. They hold up your gastrointestinal tract and act as the continence mechanism for the bladder and the urethral, anal, and vaginal orifices. Pregnancy and childbirth, straining during bowel movements, chronic coughing, being overweight, and simply the effects of gravity take a toll over the years. I remember the older women of our family back when I was a lad being concerned that they didn't "laugh too hard," when I was around, but it was only years later that I figured out why my youthful witticism was viewed with caution. (Or maybe it was just a convenient way of saying "We're watching Art Linkletter's *House Party* on the black-and-white Zenith so get lost, kid." I'll never know.)

The science is clear on this as well, and it's a happy circular relationship: sex helps strengthen the pelvic floor muscles which in turn can help you have more satisfying sex, and, as a bonus, not be as prone to stress incontinence. Sexual activity of all kinds brings healthy blood flow to the area, and orgasms are especially strengthening. A study published in the *International Urogynecological Journal* (10) and several others confirm this as one of elder life's largely unconditional WIN-WINS; women with strong pelvic floor muscles proved to have more (and more pleasurable) sex, leading to continued strong pelvic floor muscles and less incontinence.

Sex, with a partner or alone, can help you lower your risk of prostate diseases. But, only in men (Sorry, ladies). So many things are just intuitive. Common sense. You leave all that semen laying around forever without regularly flushing it out and bad things can happen to it, just like whatever was in that forgotten Tupperware bowl in the back of the refrigerator back when we were single guys.

This time we turn to a study co-authored by Lorelei Mucci, professor of epidemiology at Harvard's T. H. Chan School of Public Health. (11) Since prostate cancer is usually a malady that occurs with a long, slow progression, this study incorporated a 10-year follow-up to its original analysis and included almost 32,000 American participants. The single-sentence conclusion of the broad, complex study: "We found that men reporting higher compared to lower ejaculatory frequency in adulthood were less likely to be subsequently diagnosed with prostate cancer." Not much beating around the bush there.

Maybe that's not the best literary phrase in this context.

As with practically every aging issue, more research is needed. There are different types of prostate cancer. Some are such slow growers that we may die at 100+ still in the "watchful waiting" stage of prostate cancer, while others are fast and aggressive. Ejaculation frequency may not be equally protective against both.

But wait! There's more! Cancer isn't the only potential prostate issue that may be avoided by frequently changing the fluid. The other, even more common though less life-threatening complaint is the much bemoaned "enlarged prostate" that seems all but inevitable as men age. A study from researchers at the Mayo Clinic in Rochester, Minnesota included more than 2,000 participants and found quite clearly that men who report the most frequent ejaculations also report the lowest prevalence of moderate to severe symptoms, and consequently more positive peak urinary flow rates, smaller prostate volume, and a more positive health-related quality of life.

So, brethren, if you prefer a prostate the size of a Honda Civic instead of a Buick Electra and would rather not require a pit stop between Philly and Lancaster, we have thrown down the gauntlet.

Sex, with a partner or alone, can help improve your libido (sex drive). Use it or lose it. You already knew that about other physical functions, so why would it not apply to sex? There are many different things at play here. One is simple conditioning. Something works out well and you get rewarded, making you want it again.

I am not a golfer. Yes, that's right, I am one of the three over-50 males residing in Myrtle Beach, South Carolina who do not play golf. Ever. When I see that much grass, I would rather see a couple fat and happy Holsteins grazing it. But I have played other sports in my life, so I understand the psychological mechanism: I had a great round, either because I played well, or it was just so nice outside, or the company was good and we strengthened our bonds by doing something together, or I had that great "good tired" feeling of accomplishment afterwards. That makes me more likely to say *yes* to golfing again soon.

All of those feelings apply to having sex. Physically, it's not hard to understand: having sex increases blood flow to the genitals, enhancing lubrication and elasticity of women's vaginal tissues and oxygenating men's penile muscles, potentially leading to even better sex next time. Like that well-seasoned cast-iron skillet of grandma's: the more you use it the better it gets.

On the other hand, never lift anything heavier than a spoon with your biceps and they will become weak and flabby, making it even more difficult to lift anything heavier than a spoon in the future. You become avoidant of heavy lifting, and eventually "I don't have to" becomes "I don't want to" becomes "I can't." It's the same with sex.

This is important stuff. One of the great musical poets of our time, Stephen Stills, understands. You can't always be with the one you love, so *love the one you're with*, even if that's only *yourself*. We may hope to be Rose and Jack in the back seat of a 1912 Renault on the Titanic. But sometimes we're Ted Stroehmann "cleaning the pipes" in *There's Something About Mary*. While one sounds so much more romantic than the other, remember where that Renault ended up at the end of the film, not to mention Jack.

WHAT TO EXPECT, AND WHAT YOU CAN DO ABOUT IT

We have shown, using credible scientific sources, that sexual activity in our latter years can be beneficial to us both mentally and physically. Let's look at how our sexual functioning changes and what we can do to help ensure we still lead happy and healthy sex lives, as well as danger signs of potential serious health problems.

While our knowledge is constantly expanding, with these topics there is more "evidence suggests" than "definitely true for you," because there are so many other factors influencing our individual situations and responses.

And remember this: Everyone has his or her own moral and/or religious beliefs that affect thoughts, options, and actions about everything in general and sex in particular. You will get no "this is right and that is wrong" from me, other than a strong admonition that all sexual requests and acts be approached with respect, consent, and safety as unnegotiable ground rules. My religious denomination would have a 72-year-old widow or widower who occasionally finds physical self-pleasure on lonely evenings believe a grave sin had been committed, requiring a trip to the confessional and prayers of penance. I happen to reject that, but you do with it what you choose, applying your own standards.

Issues negatively affecting our sex lives can occur at any age, and some of these things won't happen to you or me even if we live to a hundred. Genetics and environmental factors may affect them. But many conditions are normal, natural and expected results of aging. They are nothing to be embarrassed about or ashamed of; some we just adapt to and live with, while others demand medical intervention.

Lack of sexual desire

Randall always seemed uncomfortable with talking about sex, but I finally got him to talk about it in the context of getting older and having more time to spend together. But I think I may have waited too late. I suggested "once weekly," but apparently, he understood "once, weakly" instead. I call it homonym sex. -Female (apparently an English teacher)

In both women and men, sexual desire may decline because of hormonal changes. For most of a woman's life, estrogen, chemically a steroid, is in the driver's seat when it comes to sex. With menopause, the ovaries, adrenal glands, and fat tissues that produce it go into semi-retirement. Just as you were unlikely to have distinct sexual arousal before estrogen began coursing through your veins during puberty, it can begin to decline when the spigots shut off. Women also produce a small amount of testosterone, and its demise contributes to lost desire. Often beginning a decade or so later, the same goes for men. It's unlikely anyone of either gender will have as many sexy thoughts or be so easily aroused when these hormones decline as they were when the chemicals caused utter obsession during adolescence, when nature's 'continuation of the species prime directive' was yelling *sex, sex, sex, sex* and adults in our lives were saying *no, no, no, no* for us, but not themselves.

Hurdle? Yes, there's no need pretending it isn't. It can be particularly problematic when it's more pronounced in one partner than the other, possibly leading to frustration and feelings of rejection, inadequacy, resentment, low self-esteem, and even anger. Nearly lifetime-long relationships have ended over this sad disparity. When low sex drive causes personal distress or negative relationship issues, it's called *Hypoactive Sexual Desire Disorder* and is a recognized medical problem, though not one given sufficient study or treatment, especially among the over-fifty population. It's too often just accepted as part of being around a long time, and since no one likes to think about older people getting it on anyhow, there isn't as much support for research as there is with younger subjects.

Attention research institutions and pharmaceutical companies: Performance drugs like sildenafil (Viagra) have been a multi-billion-dollar cash cow. Doesn't it make sense to pay just as much attention to *desire* as performance?

I remember, years ago, hearing two widowed aunts chatting while not knowing I was within hearing distance. Both were attractive, healthy women in their 70s. One said she really would like to find a male companion with whom to share life. "As long," she sighed, "as he wouldn't want sex. They're hard to find like that, you know." Thinking back on that now, I wonder if their lives could have been happier, healthier, and even longer had they found gentle, attentive, giving boyfriends (okay, there should be a better term, since none of us are boys or girls any longer, but what should we say? 'Male companions' sounds dull and academic) with whom to share emotional and physical relationships.

While hormonal change may be the primary reason sex drive often decreases with age, it's far from the only one. There is a long list of medications that can negatively affect sex drive. A few include anxiety and depression treatments such as SSRIs (Zoloft, Paxil, and Celexa among others), opioid pain medicines, H2 blockers (used to treat ulcers and other gastroesophageal conditions, examples famotidine, cimetidine, nizatidine and others) and chemotherapy drugs.

Unfortunately, two of the most prescribed long-term daily medications for seniors may also be culprits: statins (to lower cholesterol, such as brand name medications Lipitor, Crestor, and Zocor) and antihypertensives (to lower blood pressure).

Many of you reading this probably take one or more of those drugs. How much the medications specifically impact sex drive vs. affect sexual *performance* and secondarily your desire, or if the underlying conditions are actually the culprit, depends on the individual. Diuretics, commonly referred to in my parents' generation as "water pills," for example, can decrease blood flow to the penis even as they give the wee old guy a workout going to the bathroom more often.

Yep, I told that doctor, I said Doc, that medicine you gave me is bad for my heart. She said, bad for your heart, what do you mean? I told her it causes me to have problems in the bedroom, and it's just breaking my heart! -Male

At any age, but often increasing past fifty, things like grief from loss, depression, anxiety, and chronic physical ailments can seriously affect libido.

What you can do about decreased sex drive: As we noted above, one of best ways to boost your sexual desire is to have sex. Even if it's not epic, mind-blowing, earthmoving what-I-saw-when-I-snuck-into-*Looking for Mr. Goodbar*-in-1977 sex (Tuesday Weld was in that, as Diane Keaton's older sister. I really, really liked Tuesday Weld, just so you know. Now I am thinking about Tuesday Weld and might be all day), do *something*, with your partner or yourself, regardless of whether you reach orgasm. Even if your feel-good brain chemicals afterward can barely muster a Minnesota Lutheran "*Not bad*" instead of a Tennessee Pentecostal "*Hallelujah!*" it's worthwhile as is, and could well be aspirational, or even predictive of better things to come. Be neither ashamed nor embarrassed. Set the mood and look forward to it. You deserve it, it can make you happier, and it's good for you.

Sex starts with the brain, not the middle bits. If partnered, take an honest inventory of how often you touch one another. If you only show physical affection when interested in sex, you are expecting roasting ears without having cultivated the corn.

I grew up on a farm, by the way.

And physically, if it's card tricks or throwing darts or drawing your weapon on the firing range, exercising "muscle memory" is key. Practice makes perfect is the old saying, but we are not looking for perfect. We want to keep an important part of our identity, our humanity, our "quality of life." We want to feel pleasure, and, if partnered, want someone else to as well.

Lose the archaic embarrassment and inhibitions over talking about sex. There have been people together for a half century who have never done so. What do you like, and how? Anything new interest you? Oh, I see. Well, I really don't think I would like that, but what about a substitution?

Relaxed and unhurried, hold one another in bed naked. Rub and caress. If that's as far as you two feel like going right now, fine. You have held one another naked, rubbed, and caressed! Repeat. Repeat. Repeat. If you both honestly find that is all you desire, it's still a win! But this repeated act with no pressure may eventually lead to renewed desire for a little more, and a little more after that.

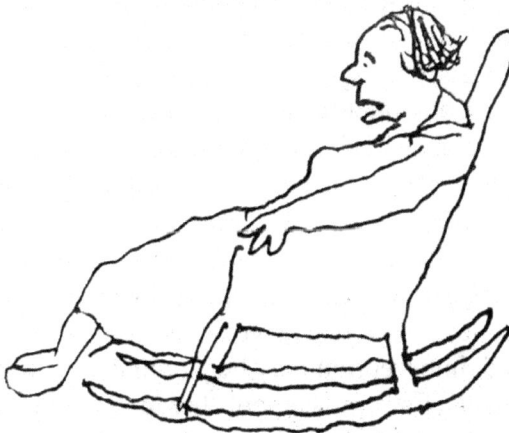

—Sigh— I used to call part of Bob my young gun. I suppose now it's Senior Staff.

Masturbate to rekindle sexual thoughts and physical feelings and to keep things working properly. Don't hide it…celebrate it! One of the things we should strive for in our golden years is self-sufficiency and not always being dependent on someone else, right? Here's your chance! Do it for, with, and to one another as well as alone whenever you feel like it. Partnered for all these years and you have never admitted, much less seen one another, indulging in self pleasure? Watch. Learn. Assist! It's good for you and your partner, both physically and psychologically.

Despite what the Beatles would have us believe in the opening track of the Abbey Road album, something always happening *together* isn't necessary. It is perfectly fine (and sometimes preferrable) to focus on one or the other partner intently without any obligation for "now it's my turn" or "at the same time" during your interlude. Maybe your turn will come tomorrow, or next week. It's not a game with a scorecard. Everyone can win, every game, but maybe not just in the same way. I will be tickled pink to help you get a *Yahtzee*, and maybe you can give me a hand with a *Large Straight* later.

Talk to your doctor about the sexual side effects of your medications. If she or he doesn't seem interested in your loss of sex drive, make the doctor listen. Be persistent. If the response is "You're old. Just get over it because it's not as important as other issues," get ye to your Find a Physician site and do just that. Find one with whom you can communicate and who will be serious about your sexual concerns, no matter your age.

Medical intervention may help, and don't be embarrassed to bring it up. Hormonal replacement therapies, for both women and men, could possibly increase sagging libido. So could treating depression, anxiety, alcoholism, and other conditions. But, like all drugs, there are side effects and cost-benefit concerns.

Hm…getting medical advice to address issues, communicating and sensuously touching your partner and/or yourself…I think I have heard of something else used to rev up sex drive, if I could just remember what it…oh, yeah. Now I remember!

YOUR OLD FRIEND PORNOGRAPHY

Things have changed so much since we were young. Cars have smaller engines, are much safer and more fuel efficient, last longer, and look like the box in which your new refrigerator was delivered. Music, as a whole, sucks in comparison to "ours." And adolescents do not lose sleep over whether their mother may find that *Playboy* magazine hidden under the mattress while cleaning. Instead, alarmingly, almost any fifth grader, if so inclined, can watch hardcore porn with three clicks on the keyboard.

So can old people, and evidently they (especially men) do just that with wild abandon. One recent extensive study of pornography use (12) is based on more than 8,000 people who participated in a survey. It found widespread pornography use across age/gender/orientation groups, including in a whopping 85.5% of men over 60, and 21% of women the same age.

The study was quite specific. It found, among senior men, fewer than 1% consumed what is considered "soft porn," while 80% watched opposite-sex partner porn, 34% same-sex partner porn, and 46% group sex porn. Among senior women, "soft porn" consumption was still less than 1%, opposite-sex partner 80%, same-sex partner 10%, and group sex 30%.

And what are our bleary old eyes watching as we tilt our heads at just the right angle to catch the bifocal? Conveniently, one of the world's largest purveyors of porn, the website Pornhub, collects such data. (You mean, they know you're watching? What a shock!) The site reports 77% of viewers are male, and the largest proportion of women watching are quite young, in the 18-24 age bracket.

The results are broken down into Categories, and Searches within those categories. For the 65+ demographic, the most popular Categories are 1. Mature, 2. Teen, 3. MILF (you can look it up for yourself if you don't know what that means because I ain't writing it here), 4. Big (penis), and 5. Lesbian. The most popular searches include, in order: Massage, Cartoon, Japanese, Granny, MILF, Stepmom, Casting, Teen, and (Fellatio). To some degree, differing interests appear to evolve as viewers age. For instance, Massage doesn't even make the top ten in the 18-24 demographic, debuts at number seven for the 25-34 set, and then steadily rises in popularity with each subsequent age group.

I was once called for jury duty, in a prosecution of a case that had an element of prostitution. During voir dire, the defense attorney asked if anyone in the potential juror pool had ever "viewed pornography." I raised my numbered paper paddle and saw another guy in front of me do the same. But then I looked around. In a courtroom full of adults, men and women of various ages, we were the only two with raised paddles. My immediate thought was not one of shame or of those copies of Penthouse sneakily passed around in my circle of buddies in high school. It wasn't even that everyone must have misunderstood the question. My thought was "Y'all lying dogs just took an oath to tell the truth, remember?" -Male

Over our long and lusty lifetimes, porn has changed. The gauzy images of beautiful people in seductive poses that still didn't necessarily satisfy adolescent curiosity about *what things actually look like* have been replaced by closeup streaming of any conceivable variation. I'm not judging, but even having been born during that narrow window of time in which one could buy a new Edsel hasn't completely burned out my "ick" receptors over the years. Just like today's marijuana isn't like yesterday's, today's porn is night-and-day different.

One of the relatively rare sex surveys including seniors was taken by Tim Rollins of *Stop Procrastinating*, an app designed to filter internet traffic, as reported in a May 28, 2021 article by Dylan Love posted on *The Daily Dot*. The survey of 2,000 men aged 50 and over revealed that 82% reported their porn habits increased because of the Internet, and 45% felt guilty about it. Marriage and family therapist Kevin Skinner has written extensively about the effect of porn on relationships, and he reports finding many women grapple with past and/or present trauma, and men struggle with compulsive behaviors and other mental health concerns like anxiety and depression. Daily porn viewing may be a symptom of the latter.

Can porn be used positively to help increase sexual desire as we age? There may be some evidence of it, with caveats. A study by Polish researchers (13) indicates porn use in adult men may have a positive impact by increasing libido and desire for a real-life partner, relieving sexual boredom, and improving sexual satisfaction by providing inspiration and motivation for real sex.

I think it's funny, but also sad in a way. My husband and I have been married for forty-five years; he has watched porn and masturbated at least occasionally the entire time, going to great lengths to hide it from me. Well, he's no better at hiding it than our son was as a teenager, though I'm sure he thinks I don't have a clue and would be mortified to "know that I know." I don't give a s---, but why does he think he has to hide something like that from me at our age? Though, come to think of it, I guess he doesn't know that I do those things as well, but I wouldn't care, unless it would make him feel inadequate somehow. It's not all about you, Phil. -Female

Soft porn has been found to relieve psychosocial stress. Creswell, Pacilio, Denson, and Satyshur found, in The Effects of a Primary Sexual Reward Manipulation on Cortisol Responses to Psychosocial Stress in Men (*Psychosomatic Medicine*, May 2013) that men who viewed mildly erotic pictures of mixed couples had lower "stress hormone" cortisol levels and did better on math tests. If only I had known THAT back when taking calculus in college!

Okay, like most guys, I look at porn sometimes, and no, I would never admit that to my wife. But just watching regular movies anymore shows what would have been porn not many years ago. I'm sure she would never consider herself as using porn, but pick up one of her romance books and read it someday. Is it really all that different, except with words instead of images? - Male

Though not as much of an issue among people our age (or at least one we are apt to admit), porn may sometimes be just plain educational. We can watch and learn, much like we do when seeking YouTube videos on how to change the battery in our car's key fob.

Researchers Taylor Kohut and William Fisher got rather specific in their study *The impact of brief exposure to sexually explicit video clips on partnered female clitoral self-stimulation, orgasm, and sexual satisfaction.* (14)

Those findings indicate *why yes, subjects orgasmed 3.51 times more often, in actual fact, thanks for asking*! Maybe there is a lesson here for us guys as well, especially ones who have been told, quite legitimately, "Good grief. Do I have to do EVERYTHING around here?" Or the infamous "Why can't you just admit you don't know where you are and ask directions?"

And, if one seeks it out, there is a growing selection of porn specifically designed to have a positive message, such as 'feminist pornography' and 'sex-positive pornography' showing consent, emphasis on mutual pleasure and caring, and diversity.

But, unfortunately, using porn to rev up your and/or your partner's interest in sex can have a downside. There is just as much research showing it can be detrimental rather than useful. It could well be a matter of type, frequency, and personality.

DANGER, GRANDPA ROBINSON! Pornography use can be an insidious substitute for the hard work of cultivating a meaningful and fulfilling sexual relationship. It can even become an obsession, preventing or harming such relationships.

My wife and I had less sex over time, and my own performance in bed when we were intimate wasn't always satisfactory. I didn't think there was any harm in secretly watching some porn to get aroused. I even thought it might help. But what happened over time was that watching porn and masturbating became so easy, so immediate, so without strings that I just stopped bothering with trying to get intimate with her. I could almost always reach orgasm, something that frustratingly wasn't reliable with her. The first time I realized there could be a problem was once when she suggested that we might shower and "cuddle in bed before we nap" one afternoon, but I declined because I had already watched porn and masturbated that morning and knew I wouldn't 'be up' to it. So, she thought I had totally lost interest in sex when in reality I was so obsessed with it that it took up a big part of my day. -Male

For seniors, there is often a vacuum left by loss of their jobs, social networks, strenuous physical activities, partners, parenting roles, and so many other things. The time and mind space will be taken up by something. It's a grand irony that many of the most positive vacuum fillers take so much effort, while the negative ones are so easy. Alcohol is easy. Isolation and inactivity in front of the television are easy.

And pornography is soooo easy. The actors in front of the camera are likely to look and act very differently than our own partner if we have one. While totally misguided, it may bring on feelings of resentment because the partner isn't like that, and self-loathing when comparing ourselves and our sex lives to that seen on the screen. Watching porn floods the brain with dopamine, but then there is the letdown, making one want to watch more porn, increasingly graphic. It can set up a classic additive sequence, a vicious cycle leaving real life sexual satisfaction drowning in its wake.

In the words of *The American Journal of Geriatric Psychology*:

"The elderly may be especially vulnerable to PIU (Problematic Internet Use) because of decreased mobility and dwindling social circles… (In) turn increased internet use might lead to diminished use of other more adaptive coping mechanisms and at the expense of deepening or maintaining real world relationships. As pornography use increases in the elderly, so does the opportunity for compulsive or impulsive use of pornography." (15)

A study published in *Behavioral Science* offers an extensive review and explanation of the subject, and there are many other studies confirming the data. Erectile dysfunction, once a non-frolicking campground inhabited by men our age, has, over the past 20 years, become more and more prevalent among younger guys, and internet porn may be at least partially to blame. (16)

The resulting article goes into brain chemistry and conditioned response models, all of which are, frankly, somewhat intuitive when you think about it. Frequent porn consumption and consequential solitary masturbation are just so much *easier* than cultivating a relationship, even one you have already been in for decades, and gives a quicker, more reliable payoff, leading to unrealistic expectations, feelings of inadequacy, resentment, and guilt.

In some cases, pornography addiction can leap off the screen and be linked to physical sex addiction. There are many stories of older men who develop porn addiction and begin emptying their coffers for prostitutes. It is not only for men, though. For example, Danielle Staub, a reality television star of *Real Housewives of New Jersey* (For the record, I don't think I have ever watched a single episode of any TV show with a title beginning with the word "Real." Even *The Real McCoys* began with "The.") has been quite honest about still struggling with sex addiction at 60.

The signs of sex addiction follow the pattern of many other addictions: You try to change your hypersexual behavior but can't seem to do so. Then you feel guilty about it, increasing your level of stress and low self-esteem, exacerbating the problem. You are preoccupied with sex, have sex with multiple random partners, your sexual behaviors become increasingly risky, other important responsibilities in your life go unfulfilled because of the time, thought, and money you put into sex. Your relationships suffer and your partner begins to complain, your sex organs become physically traumatized, or you become angry and irritable when you aren't having sex frequently.

Warning signs such as these can be applied to practically any behavior that becomes problematic. We aren't going to try to answer the "how much is too much" question. That is up to each individual and her or his partner. But, if any of those warning signs apply, be honest with yourself and seek help.

What if it doesn't directly involve another person? The American Psychological Association does not recognize Masturbation Addiction as a mental health condition in the *Diagnostic and Statistical Manual of Mental Disorders* (DSM), so when it becomes problematic, it may be referred to as a compulsion instead. Some psychologists categorize all "sex addiction" behaviors (partnered sex, porn, masturbation) as compulsions rather than true addictions. If they fit the criteria mentioned above, the distinction of categorization means little to one's everyday life.

There are people who healthily and happily masturbate every day throughout their lifetimes by choice rather than by compulsion, with no negative consequences. That same frequency for others could be considered compulsion, depending on how it affects their lives.

If you feel compulsive sexual thoughts and/or behaviors are complicating your life, seek a professional opinion. One place to start may be the Substance Abuse and Mental Health Services Administration's (a division of the U. S. Department of Health and Human Services) free 24/7, 356-days-a-year, confidential helpline. The number is 1-800-662-HELP (4357).

As your not-a-doctor, not-a-phycologist, not-a-sex-therapist guide through the world of senior sex research, I take this away from the discussion: honestly talk with your partner, if you have one, and be affectionate, responsive, and nonjudgmental. Talk with your doctor just as honestly about your level of sexual desire and compulsions. Truthfully assess your pornography use, and shift interest onto the real world. If your own level of desire is lower than your partner's, see what you can do about it, together. Take the pressure off yourself and your partner and find a way to give one another pleasure.

DECLINING PHYSICAL RESPONSES

We have spent a few thousand words talking about whether you want to have sex. Now, let's talk about *having* sex. While lack of interest tops the list when seniors are asked about what they would change about their sex lives, the below-the-neckline issues most cited include:

1. Unable to achieve orgasm
2. Experience pain during sex
3. Sex isn't pleasurable
4. Trouble lubricating
5. Anxious about performance (well, that one is both above and below the neckline, I suppose)

There they are. The Five Horsemen of the Sexual Apocalypse. Darn them!

For that information, we turned again to the work of EO Laumann and LJ Waite (Laumann EO, Waite LJ. (17)

HORSEMAN NUMBER ONE: CHASING THE BIG O

You may notice seemingly contradictory results and conclusions cited in some of the research in this section. It seems we still have much to uncover about the true nature of orgasms.

A thoroughly depressing article in *Psychology Today* by Michael Castleman (February 1, 2016) citing several large studies indicates the orgasm gender gap is huge. In heterosexual encounters, only 50-70% of women reported having orgasms, compared to 95% of men. But, as we will soon see, the news for women and all who love them gets better.

The female orgasm is, indeed, a complex (and marvelous) response. But its complexity isn't the cited reason for this gap. It's *the poor quality of the sexual stimulation women receive.*

(Brethren, do not start sending hate mail and staking out my house carrying your phallic-substitutional AK-47s. I'm just the reporter here. Look inward. Man up.)

Older research led us to believe demographics, beliefs, relationships, and histories of sexual trauma made the big difference in orgasm rates among women, and those things do matter to some extent, especially being in a positive relationship vs. just casual partners. But those factors pale in comparison to the skill and commitment of their sex partners in helping bring women to orgasm. That's of any age, and there certainly isn't any evidence to make us believe it changes significantly after we draw Social Security.

Three primary levels of sexual stimulation were considered: 1. intercourse, 2. hand massage + intercourse, and 3. hand massage + oral sex + intercourse. The difference between men and women seems stark.

For men, the orgasm rate was:
1. intercourse = 96%
2. hand massage + intercourse = 95%, and
3. hand massage + oral sex + intercourse = 98%

Well, good for you, guys. But for women:
1. intercourse = 50%
2. hand massage + intercourse = 71%, and
3. hand massage + oral sex + intercourse = 86%

Here's the good news. I mean GREAT NEWS! Even with the other complications we have talked about (and more to come), some studies show that the potential for sexual satisfaction, including the ability to orgasm, *increases* with age!

For women, that is.

A survey from *Lovehoney* with 2,100 participants found that 39% of women aged 18-25 had sex more than once a week, double the frequency of the over-45 age group. But 63% of the older women reported frequent orgasms during sex, while only 36% of the Millennials did so. Less sex, more orgasms. (18)

The contraception tracking app *Natural Cycles* surveyed 2,600 women using the standardized McCoy Female Sexuality Questionnaire methodology in 2017 and found women in the older demographic reported more satisfying sex and more frequent orgasms than younger women. Unfortunately for us, that survey didn't further break down women's ages past 36, but we like the trajectory.

Our friends across the pond asked the right questions. An article in the August 10, 2017, edition of *Carehome UK* cited, among others, a study by the International Longevity Center UK in conjunction with the University of Manchester that focused on women's sexuality as they age. Get this: the results indicate that while women's ease of arousal statistically drops post-menopause, *it can begin to rise again after age 80.* Woo hoo, Nanna!

Researchers from the University of California San Diego School of Medicine and the Veterans Affairs San Diego Healthcare System polled women who had been part of a long-term health study for almost 40 years, with a median age of 67. A robust 67.1% of respondents reported having orgasms "most of the time or always" during sex. Approximately half of the oldest women in the group (over age 80) reported sexual satisfaction (including arousal, lubrication, and orgasm) "almost always or always." This was despite a reported overall decline in sexual desire.

"But it still beats the heck out of canasta," one respondent volunteered. (Okay, I made that up, but I really hope someone said it.)

Think back to the analogy I made at the beginning of this chapter. Most people may not have a great desire to go to the gym, but they know it's good for them, and end up enjoying it at least a little and feeling good about being there.

There are so many other emotional and physical factors involved, but the real key to female orgasm, no matter one's age, is quality of stimulation. As women age, their partner's or their own solo strategies can become more experienced and knowledgeable about how to bring effective stimulation. There may finally be time and motivation to find out exactly what is it that gets you over the top. That can, with communication and patience and willingness, be explored with a partner, but sometimes most efficiently alone, focused solely on oneself, perhaps trying out toys as well as techniques.

As we saw in the first study cited in this section, intercourse alone doesn't cut it. Manual stimulation and oral sex, especially when patiently guided with open communication, may bring older women to that illusive *best sex ever.*

My husband has always wanted oral sex, but it just doesn't appeal to me, so I never go all the way with it, and it probably does disappoint him. I used to fake orgasm during intercourse, but the only way I really reach it is when he gives ME oral sex. I need that direct stimulation in just the right place, and it can be very good. He seems to enjoy it, too, but I suspect he wishes it were reciprocated. I suppose there is some inequity in all that, but we don't really feel comfortable discussing specifics. -Female

Remember: for women, hand massage + oral sex + intercourse = 86%.

Now we will turn to aging male orgasm, where the science isn't quite so rosy.

With men, of course, the questions of "did I have an orgasm, or didn't I?" or "is he faking it" are less of an issue. Under most circumstances (I had to spell check that word in this context) there is evidence of ejaculation. There's semen *somewhere.*

There are a few exceptions, in the form of dry orgasms. It's not uncommon for an adolescent male's first orgasm or two to lack ejaculation, or for that first ejaculation to come while the lad is asleep, much to his waking alarm. (When I taught high school anatomy and physiology years ago, I advised my students that not forewarning their someday sons about nocturnal emissions was just as poor a parenting practice as not forewarning their someday daughters about the onset of menstruation. You may *tut tut*, but think about it.) Males also have a refractory period in which more semen is produced, and if one orgasms soon again before the reservoir is refilled it may be without ejaculation.

But orgasm without ejaculation among seniors will likely be of two types: for whatever reason there is no semen reserve, or the semen goes backwards into the bladder instead of springing out into the world and joining the party via the penis. The latter is called *retrograde ejaculation*, and it's not a good thing.

There can be several causes. Retrograde ejaculation can be a warning sign of prostate problems or nerve damage due to diabetes or stroke or MS. It's common for men to be able to orgasm but not ejaculate after having prostate surgery or radiation treatment. Other times there can be a blocked sperm duct.

If you have dry orgasms other than on the rare occasion that you are having a second one so soon that your body hasn't had a chance to refill the tank (you old horn dog, you!), see your doctor and be both candid and complete in your descriptions. She will order urine and blood tests and perhaps an ultrasound. Because it could be the sign of something important, don't delay.

Even if things move in the right direction, there is just no denying it: unlike women, as men age, it will become harder to have an orgasm. Get used to it. But *how* you get used to it is key.

It's not just aging, either. Many medications affect the ability to reach orgasm. Many of the same meds that affect libido (such as SSRIs) are notorious for preventing or delaying male orgasm. In fact, they are sometimes prescribed to combat premature ejaculation. That is where, I assume, the fine line between doses that *delay* vs. *prevent* is an important one. Opiate pain medications and alcohol may also prevent or delay orgasm, if they even allow the subject to get an erection in the first place. Being able to maintain an erection but going a frustratingly long time being stimulated without climaxing (which, when one was younger, might have sounded intriguing without the word *frustratingly*), or *delayed ejaculation* is less frequently reported in older men than its opposite malady, premature ejaculation. Realistically, many older men will lose their erection before an ejaculation becomes significantly delayed, moving it into the category of erectile dysfunction instead.

Yet another possibility is being able to orgasm, but the ejaculation being very weak. Those old muscles are just going to produce a dribble of semen instead of forcefully ejecting it.

In other words, no more "Hey kid, you'll put your eye out with that thing!"

Over time, the penis may require more, and more direct, stimulation to bring you to orgasm. Our advice is like that for women: find out what it takes, alone or with patient assistance, and do it. But there are some things to remember about that advice.

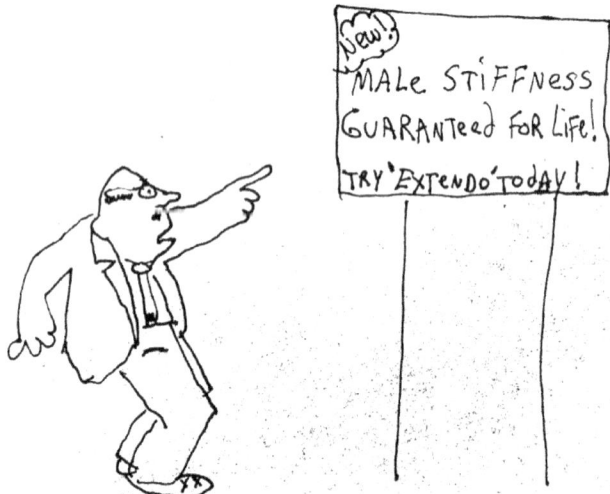

Especially with male orgasms, there may need to be a balance between quantity and quality. We have a longer refractory period than women, in general. The once-a-week orgasm may well be more intense than the daily orgasm. While priming the pump of sexual desire and keeping everything in working order is important for both sexes, there is something to be said for a period of anticipation, perhaps with sexual stimulation not taken as far as orgasm, and sex toys can be helpful.

How much anticipation? We have already determined that sex, and having orgasms, is healthy for both women and men. It strengthens muscles and keeps them healthy, helps you sleep, releases endorphins, reduces stress, burns a couple calories, and lots of good things. But are there delayed orgasmic benefits to periods of abstinence, especially for men? That's the premise of pundits, primarily on the far right, promoting what they call *No Nut November,* which was originally intended to be satirical, I believe, but grew into an actual thing. Proponents claim improved sex lives, feelings of self-confidence and control, higher bowling scores, etc.

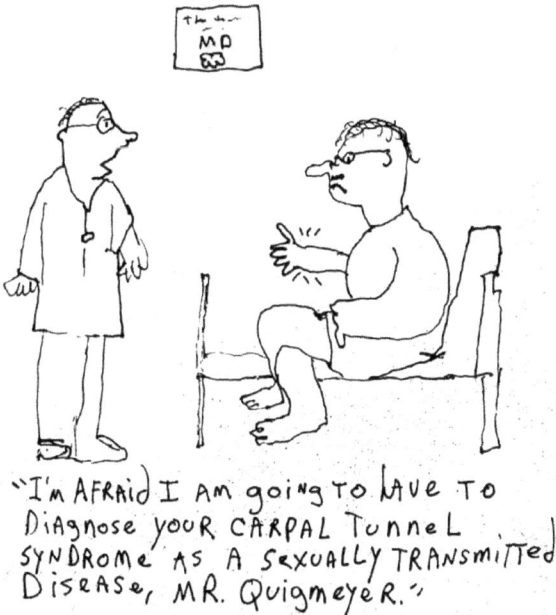

"I'm AFRAid I AM going To HAve To Diagnose your CARPAL Tunnel SYNDRome AS A SexuaLLy TRANsmiTTed Disease, MR. Quigmeyer."

I say, show me the science. And come on, I already do Dry January. Isn't that enough? But, if you ejaculate frequently, waiting awhile until the next one could increase its intensity, with no harm done. Some guys spend a lifetime chasing the elusive technique known as "edging," which entails stimulation (solo or partnered) right up to the point of inevitable ejaculation, then abruptly ending the stimulation just long enough to avoid climax before resuming, supposedly leading to an intense orgasm when it finally arrives. Considering the mandatory refractory period, this may be as close as men can get to the Nirvana of multiple orgasms available to women but may also require practice and skill. But, hey, if you have time on your hands…so to speak?

Many men respond to prostate massage with intense orgasms. Whether this is done solo or partnered is much like any other sexual practice: your business. Some men dislike the sensation of an object being inserted into their rectum to stimulate their prostate, while others report enjoying it immensely. There is some evidence that prostate massage orgasms require a shorter refractory time than the regular kind.

Common sense should prevail. If using a finger instead of an inanimate object, you or your partner should trim those fingernails. Perhaps consider timing, having had your daily bowel movement already. There's nothing wrong with using surgical gloves. Go slow, be gentle, and always use a lubricant (more on those later).

And the cautions: Afterwards, of course, wash and sanitize everything. If using an object instead of a finger, make sure it's of a shape that it doesn't cause damage or *get lost*.

Yes, that happens, and evidently often enough to warrant a medical diagnosis: *RFOs*, or Rectal Foreign Objects. Some of the objects presented in emergency rooms include plastic and glass bottles, cucumbers, carrots, deodorant containers, candles, and, of course, dildos and vibrators. Even light bulbs have made their way into the dark. This can be serious stuff, requiring surgery. Many sufferers delay going to the doctor and may employ dangerous methods to try to retrieve the object themselves due to embarrassment ("I, um, just got out of the shower and accidently sat on this zucchini from the garden, Doc. You know how it is when they come in all at once and they're everywhere.") But those measures and delaying treatment can lead to rectal perforation, peritonitis, hypovolemic shock, thrombosed hemorrhoids, and other dangerous complications.

So, you heard it here first, friends: For prostate massage, use your finger, borrow one from a friend, or use a specifically designed sex toy with a flange or handle sufficient to keep it from being inserted too far.

Caution number two: I hope you all (well, not the women readers) have an annual prostate exam. If there is any sign of prostate cancer (you haven't had an exam in too long, or you have an elevated PSA, or you like so many are in the "watchful waiting" stage), it is best to avoid prostate massage, regardless of your orgasm pursuit. It can cause cancer cells to separate and spread to nearby tissues. It's not worth it.

FOR BOTH WOMEN AND MEN: Who doesn't love a good orgasm? Like spaghetti, there are only two kinds, good and better. You may occasionally have it at Sardis, but still really appreciate Chef Boyardee from a can if that's what is immediately available.

But, if achieving orgasm (a term common in the literature, but one I dislike…it makes it sound like 'achievement' is an all-or-nothing proposition with a possibility of failure. This is a situation in which the much maligned "participation trophy" concept is perfectly valid!) is your sole reason for sex, either solo or partnered, you may be missing the point. We've spent our lives being so goal oriented that we are intent on a specific result instead of pleasure and connection. Reread the first paragraph of this and every chapter. If we are so focused on "getting there" at the expense of enjoying "being *here*," we may be full of regret when "here" runs out.

Whew. Having been at my computer up to my eyeballs in old people's orgasms for some time now, I know more than I did, but there is little I will feel comfortable dropping into conversation at my next book club meeting while helping set up the refreshments. But, in a nutshell:

Research into senior sexual desire and orgasm is sparse, and results sometimes inconsistent, but most of it indicates women may desire sex less as they age but may still have sex frequently and enjoy it even more than when they were younger. The key is learning what it takes, and that is often slow, steady, and direct clitoral stimulation through hand massage and oral sex instead of relying solely on intercourse. Self-stimulation and use of sex toys along with patient coaching of one's partner (if present) are the keys.

On the other hand, men's orgasms are likely to be fewer and more difficult to reach as we age. But the same advice (self-stimulation, massage, toys) along with that all-important patient coaching of one's partner (if present) is just as valid.

Lose the emphasis on the all-important Big O. It's the journey, not the destination, that's important.

HORSEMEN NUMBERS TWO, THREE, AND FOUR: IT SHOULD FEEL GOOD

Experience pain during sex, Sex isn't pleasurable, and Trouble lubricating: We know we can all probably name several things that weren't painful at age 18 but are now. Sex shouldn't be one of them.

Painful vaginal sex is called *dyspareunia*, and surveys of postmenopausal women who are not on hormone replacement therapy estimate that from 20% to 30% of women experience it. One of the main culprits is the change in vaginal tissue brought about by decreased estrogen levels, including the tissue becoming thinner and less elastic. There's simply less cushion for the pushin'. Sometimes other factors, such as damage from childbirth or infections, can cause pain during sex. There can also be involuntary vaginal wall spasms (vaginismus) that essentially close the vagina and prevent penetration. Causes can be either physiological or psychological, such as stress, fear of intimacy, relationship issues, or concerns over body image. One of the most common complaints is vaginal dryness.

Fortunately, things can be done to ease all these concerns. An excellent source for understanding what's going on and what can be done (men, do not skip this!) is an article by Dana Sparks adapted from a piece in the *Mayo Clinic Health Letter* by Dr. Beatriz Stamps of the Gynecology Department of the Mayo Clinic, Phoenix branch.

First step: this is something you need to talk about with your doctor and do so candidly. Painful sex can be a symptom of serious conditions that require intervention. But often, simple treatments and/or techniques can help.

As estrogen dissipates with menopause, so does the vagina's natural moisture. That moisture serves more purposes than sexual lubrication, keeping the walls healthy, warding off bacteria, and avoiding itching and pain during urination. One way to kickstart the body's natural production of vaginal lubrication is to return small doses of the hormone right to the front line, in the form of topical estrogen treatments. These come in various forms, including a tablet or soft gel inserted into the vagina (daily at first, then less often, such as twice weekly), a slow-release hormone ring (one ring inserted into the vagina and lasting about three months, perhaps long enough to be referred to as *my precious*), and a cream delivered through an applicator. Unlike just using a lubricant when needed, these treatments can reverse the vaginal changes brought about by menopause. And yes, one can have sex with the tablets or rings in place.

What about more systemic hormonal replacement by simply taking a pill? Talk to your doctor, because that kind of broad hormonal replacement may come with increased risks and is not as widely used as it once was for that reason.

Now, to a therapy less costly and hopefully more pleasurable: strengthening the vaginal and pelvic floor muscles. Like any other muscle, the more it's exercised, the more toned it becomes. Go to the gym and lift weights, and at first your arm muscles will ache, but after a while, they become stronger, and you can lift the same weight without the pain. Vaginal muscles are also *muscles* and respond in kind. If nothing has penetrated your vagina to exercise those muscles and increase blood flow in years, then it's no surprise that workout sessions will be difficult at first.

When you go to the gym, it's not your gym partner's responsibility to make sure your biceps get a workout. Sure, he or she can spot you with the free weights, but the ultimate responsibility is yours. So, if frequent vaginal exercise comes about by insertion of your partner's penis and/or fingers and that's what satisfies you, wonderful. If you need to supplement that, it's not difficult. Your own fingers or sex toys can do the trick. Just remember that, like any other muscle tone, it dissipates all too quickly if not consistently flexed. Use it, meet *lose it*.

A simple vibrator, readily available and inexpensive, may be sufficient. Make sure it's big enough to be fully inserted without losing it, instead of a very small one designed to only be used on the clitoris. There's nothing wrong with having one of those as well, of course, but the two sizes have different functions. While there is little danger of an object being "stuck" in the same sense as in the rectum (squatting and bearing down will usually push the object back toward the opening), it can still be distressing.

In some cases, medical devices called *vaginal dilators* are recommended. They come in different diameters so one can start small and work up as the muscles become healthier. I am sure there are cases in which they serve a very specific purpose that could not be as efficiently accomplished with other devices, or even regular, enjoyable sex. But, when reading the instructions, I am not sure, other than the specifically graduated diameters, of the difference between using these and the less clinical (and expensive) dildo (static) or vibrator (active) or your own or a partner's body parts:

Apply a water-based lubricant. Lay in a comfortable position on your back with legs bent at the knees. Insert until you feel tension. Move dilator around inside your vagina, using a circular motion, then a slow thrusting motion. Gently remove after 15 minutes. Thoroughly clean. Over time, aim for a larger diameter and deeper penetration. (Adapted from information on the use of vaginal dilators provided by The Cleveland Clinic)

I mean...yeah. Sounds good to me. The only things missing from the instructions are scented candles and Barry White's *Can't Get Enough* album on continuous play in the background. Most of us guys are trainable enough (I hope) to take great interest in assisting with the delicate procedure. Don't you wish all medical instructions were this intriguing? "Well, it's doctor's orders, so I guess I had better get to it." (More on sex toys later)

Another way to help strengthen the vaginal muscles is do Kegel exercises, which are free, easy, and effective. They can even be beneficial for men's sexual and urological health as well. Imagine stopping and then restarting your urine stream, or that you are trying to keep yourself from passing gas. Those are the muscles you want to practice flexing. To be sure, insert a finger into your vagina and tighten and release your muscles. A good regimen is to make sure your bladder is empty and sit or lie down. Tighten for five seconds, then relax for five seconds, and repeat ten times, three times a day. It might take a month or longer, but they should make a difference. Unlike some other exercises, Kegels aren't necessarily in the "more is better" category, since increasing them can lead to muscles so toned that they could inhibit penetration or urination. Think big biceps in a snug t-shirt.

Kegel exercises for men use basically the same instructions, but with a finger in the anus to make sure they have identified the correct muscles.

It's less common for sex to be painful for men. A swollen prostate can cause some pain in the rectum or internal area between anus and scrotum after ejaculation, but it's usually fleeting. Taking a warm bath or literally "walking it off" usually suffices. If more pronounced, it could be a symptom of prostatitis. More often, friction can be a source of pain for men, as well as for women. This brings us to our next topic:

LUBE, GLORIOUS LUBE: It's unfortunate that masturbation, lubrication, and sex toys are such uncomfortable topics for some of us, but we must acknowledge they are, even for me, having grown up in a typical 60s-70s household where sex, in any form, was a taboo topic, unless it was approached with scorn, shame, embarrassment, and ridicule. Sadly, many of you can relate, I'm sure. If we are going to enjoy the health and happiness benefits of sex while we age, all these things need to be part of the discussion.

Post menopause, women can expect to produce less natural vaginal lubrication, both the always-present kind and the increased wetness during sexual arousal. With insufficient slick and slippery natural moisture, penetration of a penis, finger, or sex toy hurts.

The default strategy doesn't even require a trip to the drug store. A happily sufficient wetness can often be found simply by extending foreplay before attempting penetration. Up the kissing and caressing stage. Gently massage the labia before spreading it, then begin with the clitoris, where so much female sexual satisfaction and orgasmic possibility may be gained. Many women prefer slow, circular, consistent clitoral massage (hand or vibrator), while many guys, using what works best on their own sex organ as a guide, may mistakenly opt for the "harder, faster, stronger" approach. It's an individual preference and communicating what you want is crucial. Then move on to unhurried oral sex. More time and patience and pleasure spent there will often make insufficient lubrication a moot point when it's time (if desired) for penetration.

Journey, not destination.

But in some cases, natural lubrication just isn't going to be sufficient, and even clitoral touching will be uncomfortable if the area is too dry. Having a Plan B (and I am not talking about contraception…sooo past that!) already in hand, or at least in the nightstand drawer, is always a good idea. Buy some lube and give it a test run even if you don't quite need it yet.

What kind? Like deciding on new flooring for the foyer, the decision is complicated by having such a wide variety of choices. (Do you ever long for the old days when there was one phone company?) Walk down the motor oil aisle at your local auto parts store and you will be faced with just about the same bombardment of lubrication decision making. Here are the basics:

Water-based lubricants don't last particularly long, but, depending on circumstances, may not need to do so. They won't cause harm to condoms or sex toys.

Silicone lubricants last longer and are also compatible with condoms but could damage certain sex toys.

Hybrid lubricants are a blend of the two, with some characteristics of each.

Also used since time began: Food oils (when I was in my early 20s, I was at a party with people mostly older than me, and the conversation began to lag. "I guess it's time to break out the Wesson oil" one wag quipped. I assumed we were moving to the kitchen to make that Appalachian delicacy, fried apple pies). Nothing new here. The earliest mention of olive oil being used as a sexual lubricant I find is from Greece in 350 BC, for use with their padded leather dildos. Folks in ancient Japan extracted lube from seaweed and yams. While harmless for male masturbation I suppose, food oils shouldn't be used for intercourse, as they can sometimes lead to bacterial or yeast infections. Some folks swear by coconut and olive oils, but be cautious.

Petroleum-based lubricants (If that same wag had said "break out the Vaseline" I would have gotten the drift, but still not have been amused) shouldn't be used internally because they can irritate and lead to infections. They can also break down condoms.

How to choose? For vaginal penetration, a pH between 3.8 and 4.5 is preferable, analogous to the environment. Another potential factor is known as "high osmolality," or how much moisture they draw from surrounding tissue. The World Health Organization has even weighed in on this, recommending osmolality less than 380 mOsm/kg. (19) Fascinating reading...I do it so you don't have to!

Additives can be of concern. In *Prevention Magazine* (October 5, 2016), Kelli Acciardo cites various research sources that suggest avoiding a host of chemicals found in personal lubricants, including glycerin, petrochemicals such as propylene glycol, and polyethylene glycol (we aren't trying to keep our radiator from freezing in the bedroom, now are we?), preservatives like parabens, benzyl alcohol, citric acid, and benzocaine. Plus, "artificial flavorings and preservatives" in general, whether in food or lube, should give us pause.

I'm not giving brand recommendations, but for that you have lots of info to help with your choices. Apply lube to your or your partner's fingers and to your clitoris and vagina during foreplay, and your male partner can apply some (or better still, you do it for him) to his penis before intercourse if desired.

As we have noted, attempted intercourse with insufficient lubrication can be painful for both women and their male partners. Outside of that, for guys the conversation shifts from the internal to the external and will lead to discussion of a little-discussed male sex problem.

Stroking the penis dry vs. stroking it with a lubricant, whether done solo or by a partner, are two very different sensations

(I'm told). Using lube more closely approximates the feeling of vaginal intercourse and prevents the penis from becoming chaffed, even to the point of micro-tears in the skin. To have a partner use a slow, slippery hand to bring a guy to full arousal or all the way to climax is a very intimate and sensual experience that can sometimes help achieve orgasm when vaginal penetration does not.

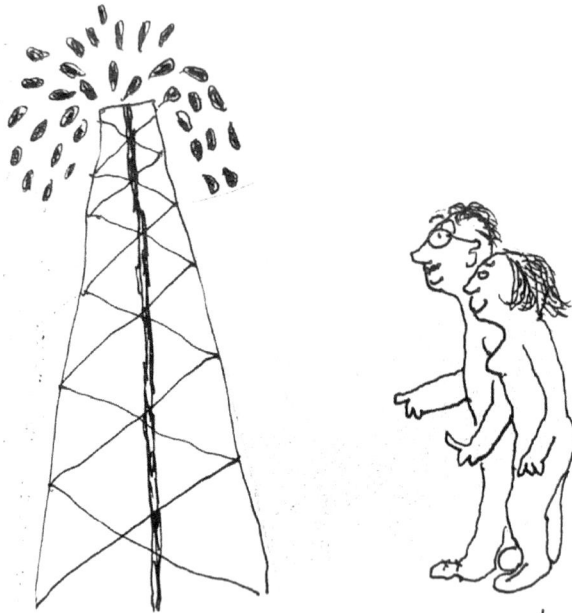

IT'S LuBe, HerB. We've STRucK LuBe!

Now a little-discussed problem: a good reason for men to use lube when masturbating is to avoid the condition known as *Idiosyncratic Masturbatory Syndrome* (or *Style*) (IMS), often referred to with a term supposedly coined by sex journalist Dan Savage, DEATH GRIP. Simply put, guys masturbate in a certain way, often with a firm grip and increasing speed and vigor and get used to that sensation to reach orgasm. Then, when having sex with a partner, her hand, vagina, or mouth do not match those speed and pressure parameters, making the bloke frustrated to the point of not only failing to reach orgasm, but losing his erection entirely.

There's nothing funny about that scenario. If the guy blames himself, there can be guilt and a sense of shame and failure and performance anxiety, making things even worse. But the darkest of the dark side is that sometimes the guy will then blame his partner for not arousing him sufficiently.

Arriving at Death Grip is usually a long journey. As adolescents, most guys do not live in households so open about sexuality that they are encouraged to masturbate in the healthiest way possible and provided lube. Does that describe your family? Instead, it is done stealthily, secretively, and swiftly for fear of getting caught. Eventually the penis begins to become desensitized; the grip tightens and the speed increases to compensate.

You don't have to be a senior citizen for this to become a problem. While communication about how to pleasure one another is vitally important, it may be unrealistic to expect your partner to become adept in exactly reproducing your idiosyncratic style. You may be a candidate for a Death Grip Reset.

During the reset, you might consider reducing your masturbatory frequency, but feel free to (preferably with the help of a partner) gently stimulate your penis, enough for arousal but not to orgasm. No firm stroking, and use lube. When alone, always use lube, gentle and slow motions, and maybe change hands. In fact, even breaking the hand/penis muscle memory relationship completely may be beneficial, and battery-operated "handsfree" masturbators may help accomplish that mission if a willing partner isn't available. It will feel awkward at first and you may become frustrated and tempted to grab-and-go like you have for decades.

It will take time but be worth it. The condition does not get enough attention from urologists or therapists, and there should be more research into ways to mitigate it. Maybe it's time to bring public attention to bear and raise research funds, But how? *I know!* A Death Grip telethon, airing annually on February 15 to pick up the pieces after a disappointing St. Valentine's Day. I wonder where it should air? (cough-FoxNewsChannel-cough).

GIRLS AND BOYS AND THEIR TOYS: Now that we're all lubed up and our pelvic walls are strong and handsome while our grip is sensitive and sustaining instead of deadly, it's time to talk about a happier topic. Since we were wee tots, we've loved toys! Johnny West with all those accessories, still in the box…how I wish Mom hadn't thrown them out.

Whether or not you use sex toys, alone or with your partner, is your business. But from one senior to another: if you don't, you could be unnecessarily missing out on a lot of pleasure, just because of the fear of trying something new or the baggage of outdated thinking.

We had gone away for the weekend just before Christmas and were having drinks at a nice bar. I checked my email and saw the sex toys I ordered had arrived at our home, so I told my wife they would be awaiting us. She didn't believe me that I had ordered sex toys. In fact, she bet me $50 that I was kidding! Easiest $50 I've ever made, and we've used them several times since. But I was so nervous about doing it that, had we not been having drinks, I'm not sure I would have mustered the courage to even tell her about them. –Male

Start with a simple, versatile vibrator. Solo or with your partner, run it along your body, including nipples, on low speed. Ease it around the labia or the underside of the penis and perineum. Gently massage the (properly moist) clitoris. A slow, consistent circular motion in either of these places can sometimes bring about intense orgasm, or alternatively just plain feel darned good and heighten your arousal. When ready, gently insert it. If new to the practice, go slowly. Savor the sensation. Women may enjoy the type of vibrator that is angled upward to hit the "G-spot" (Like Shangri-la, there's still controversy over its existence, I know) while a smaller part at roughly a right angle also massages the clitoris. Think about your partner gently using this dual-purpose thingy on you while kissing your chest and…

Ahem. You get the point. It can stimulate guys just as effectively, as can silicone sleeves that approximate the structure of a vagina (use lube), and even the "handsfree" devices that fit on the penis and stimulate the underside of the glans. You may also try a rubber ring with a tiny vibrating motor that fits snugly around the base of the penis, aiding in arousal.

With your partner, or alone, these can add pleasure to your sex life and even help reach orgasm when it may be otherwise difficult.

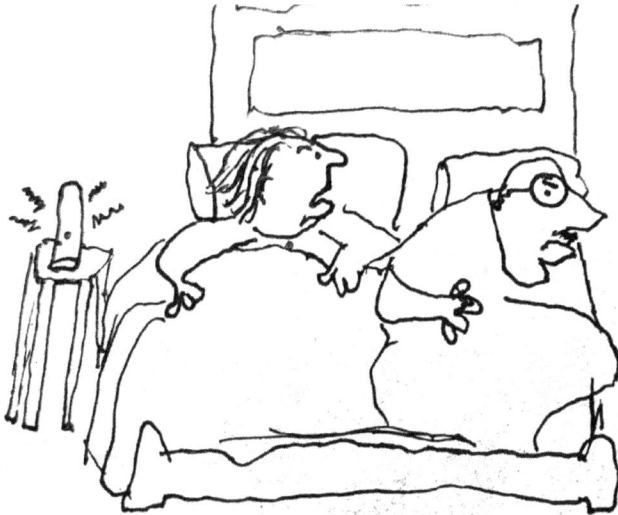

NO, RAYMOND, YOU CAN'T TAKE MY
BATTERIES FOR YOUR TV REMOTE!

There are a hundred variations of basic sex toys. You no longer have to risk being seen going into a sex shop to see them, since, like everything else, they can be ordered online. (I know that's convenient, but I do worry about the future of brick-and-mortar retail for just about everything, don't you? Chances are you bought this book online instead of at a bookstore where you could sit and read with a cup of coffee. We will miss those when they're gone, mark my word.)

Is there a downside? It goes without saying that sex toys are to be kept scrupulously clean and sanitary, and not used with a parade of different partners or put places they shouldn't after being in, well, certain other places. That's common sense, as is always being gentle in their use. If something hurts, stop it. Make sure your chosen toy doesn't contain any toxic chemicals and watch out for allergic reactions.

What about becoming addicted to your sex toys? In an article by Zahra Barnes published in *Self Magazine* (January 15, 2016), Dr. Mary Jane Minkin, clinical professor of OBGYN at Yale Medical School, says it's unlikely. Your clitoris may become desensitized for a time with vigorous use, but it's usually temporary. You can overdo almost any good thing, right? But she does recommend changing things up, so you aren't repeating exactly the same action every time. Don't become so conditioned. Maybe your partner can help with that! It's the same for men. While using a vibrator may not become as detrimental as Death Grip, changing things up will keep the wee fellow from becoming so accustomed to getting exactly what he wants that he pouts at anything different.

Do yourself and your partner a favor. Talk about what you would like to try and then go shopping.

BUT BAD SEX THINGS CAN STILL HAPPEN: You know all those scary things that were thrown at you as reasons to not have sex back when you were young? I hate to tell you, but except for pregnancy (assuming post-menopausal women), they're all still out there now. Yes, we can still get STDs, even at our advanced age. In fact, according to the Centers for Disease Control and Prevention (HIV, Hepatitis, STD, TB, *Social Determines of Health Data*, 2018) the rate of STDs has more than doubled in the past decade among Americans 65 and older.

More…than…doubled. In ten years. Let that sink in. Researchers in an extensive study cite various causes, including a lack of knowledge and communication with doctors and partners, a reduced public health emphasis on safe sex practices among seniors, and lack of screening in our age group. (21)

In our minds, we may be the same rebels who were adolescents back when music was great and may still have a "it won't happen to me" attitude, now laced with "if it ain't happened yet, it ain't happening now" and tinged with "what the heck, I may not have long left anyhow." Pardon my soapbox, but I read stupidity and a callous, dangerous disregard for others in those sentiments.

"You and grandma doing okay, grandpa?" "Oh, not bad for our age. This shoulder that I hurt years ago bothers me sometimes, especially when it rains, and between your grandma and me, we have bacterial vaginosis, chlamydia, gonorrhea, hepatitis, herpes, HIV, HPV, PID, syphilis and trichomoniasis flareups now and then. I guess we should be more careful. Always should have."

No, it's not funny. Educate yourself. We live in the instant information age. If you are having sex with someone other than an exclusive long-term partner, use condoms and dental dams, and practice other safe sex techniques. If you have had unprotected sex with a new partner, get tested for STDs, including HIV. I don't know a soul of any age who would rather have a conversation about sexual history than *have sex*, but do it, no matter how much of an embarrassing buzzkill it may be.

If these things can ruin the lives of the young and healthy, what do you think they can do to your tired old immune system? And remember something I wish were never again an issue: consent. No means no, stop means stop, and nobody owes you *anything* or is obligated to do *anything* when it comes to her or his own body. Period. We're better than that. And if it wasn't in your cultural background to speak up about what you do or don't want sexually throughout your life, this is one area above almost any other in which you must learn a new skill. If there have been a hundred enthusiastic yeses in the past, even with the same partner, tonight's *no* is just as valid as ever.

HORSEMAN FIVE: ANXIOUS ABOUT PERFORMANCE:

I am happy my wife and I still have sex, but it follows a predictable routine that has become so stressful that I find excuses to not do it. I pleasure her first, and I enjoy caressing and masturbating her. She's responsive to it. Then I bring her to orgasm with oral sex, but when I enter her I almost always lose my erection before I climax. The threat of it makes me want to go faster before I lose it, but she likes it slower, so I slow down and then lose it before finishing. I give up and roll off. I'm frustrated. She's frustrated.

Later, while she's in the shower, I will bring myself to orgasm, which I can usually accomplish. -Male

I remarried in my 50s after my first wife passed. I wasn't anxious about performance, I was petrified! And not in the "turned to stone" sense of the word if you get my drift. It took quite a while to figure out that, in addition to all the other things swirling around one's mind about a new relationship, I subconsciously felt guilt that I was somehow being unfaithful to my deceased wife, something I had never been. It's gotten better, but the initial anxiety early in my new marriage has stuck with me. -Male.

You knew we would get to erectile dysfunction eventually. In this chapter, I mean. It's a self-fulfilling prophecy for many men: you are anxious about your sexual performance because of past failures, which causes the stress response which in turn causes erectile dysfunction or a failure to orgasm, leading to more stress and anxiety next time, or avoiding sex altogether.

I figure a guy's given just so many good hard-ons in his lifetime, and I've about used mine up, I reckon. – Male

There are so many things that can affect erections other than just age. A few common medications can lead to ED, such as diuretics, antihypertensives, antihistamines, antidepressants, Parkinson's disease treatments, antiarrhythmics, tranquilizers, muscle relaxants, nonsteroidal anti-inflammatory drugs, statins, histamine H2-receptor antagonists, hormones, chemotherapy medications, prostate cancer drugs, opioid pain medications, anti-seizure medications…did I say a *few*? Plus, the conditions these drugs are meant to treat, such as diabetes, heart disease, depression, and many others can cause ED as well. Then there are all those things we bring on ourselves through using alcohol, illegal drugs, and smoking, plus nervousness, fatigue, general stress, lack of self-confidence with your partner, relationship concerns…the list goes on and on. It's almost a wonder any of us can ever rise up to pay the matter full attention.

While the first defense against flagging out seems to be a pill these days, there are other strategies. One is a vacuum pump. Simply fit the cylinder over your penis and pump it up. The vacuum draws blood into the penis. Then put a rubber band around the base to keep the blood in place, for up to a half hour. There are also prescription injections, administered with a tiny needle, right into the side of the penis. The thought is probably worse that the actual shot.

In more severe cases, a penile implant consisting of inflatable cylinders can be surgically installed. There is a reservoir of fluid placed under the abdominal muscles, and the pump is inside the scrotum. You literally pump yourself up. When finished, press a valve to return to flaccidity. (I think that's the first time I have ever written that word.)

When the first effective ED medications in pill form hit the market, the world changed. The four most prescribed are avanafil, sildenafil (Viagra), tadalafil (Cialis), and vardenafil. Be sure your doctor knows if you are taking nitrate medications, alpha-blockers, or enzyme blockers before accepting a prescription for any of these drugs.

Many men who are prescribed these drugs (and there are millions of prescriptions each year) end up disappointed. That may be because they expected a miracle. Without arousal, drugs do not "give you" an erection at all, much less the erection of a 16-year-old during the Memorial Day weekend pool opening. The drugs work best on an empty stomach, and take a while to kick in. A lot of guys eventually even give up on ED meds. A study of 14,370 men found the main reasons given were that the treatment didn't work, cost too much, had unacceptable side effects, or the men simply lost interest in sexual relationships. (21)

Talk to your doctor. I say that a lot, and for good reason. ED meds may or may not be for you; they may or may not even *work* for you. If you do try the ED drugs, give them a chance, and manage your expectations. They do not affect sexual desire, except perhaps by bolstering your self-confidence, though that, in itself, may be worthwhile.

A note to partners: I cannot speak for all men, of course, but being in possession of at least a bit of male ego, I advise against asking "Did you remember to take your pill?" While a perfectly valid question, it could be a downer, implying you are more interested in the quality of his erection than of your chance for intimacy no matter what form it takes.

Getting a satisfactory erection isn't the whole ballgame, of course. Here I'm reminded of something supposedly said by my favorite Founding Father Ben Franklin when asked what kind of government we would have. "A republic, if you can keep it." Old Ben was quite a wag, and I can channel him in this context, "An erection, if you can keep it." It's not just having one, it's what you do with it later that counts.

That leaves guys with a rather Goldilocksian path: this climax is too fast (premature ejaculation, PE). This climax is too slow (delayed ejaculation, DE). Or, this climax is juuuust right.

With men, performance anxiety is closely tied to sexual response. For women, it can be associated with body image concerns. Not one of us look like we did in our 20s, and, especially with women, unrealistic body image standards have been the societal and cultural yoke under which our generation toiled. Compared to men, the double standard is enormous.

It's a vicious circle, I guess. She's not interested in having sex because she says I never touch her unless I want sex. But any time I touch her, the thought that we don't have sex comes bounding into my brain and I think 'So, she thinks I'm good enough to cuddle her but not good enough to make love to her' and I pull away. And so it continues, neither of us getting what we want, and both staying ticked off about it. – Male

The goal should be to stay as fit and healthy as possible. If you want to try all those things available to help you "look younger" and that makes you feel better, have at it. But ask yourself, "Am I doing this for me? Do I feel better about myself with this injection, coloring, cosmetic surgery, etc.?" If the answer is yes, that's wonderful. But if it's solely for someone else's gratification, maybe it's time to evaluate your priorities. Life is too short to always focus on someone else, especially when it comes to your body. You know what brings you pleasure and peace; that's what is important and carries over into the bedroom. If your partner doesn't see beauty in your body and is not attracted to it, there may be bigger relationship issues than sex afoot that demand attention.

Have an honest discussion about it. People can learn together. People can change *together*. If they choose to do neither, they can also be jettisoned.

After discussing so many physical factors that affect aging sex lives, remember that now, just as when we were younger, the most important sex organ is the brain. Our expectations, our clinging embarrassment or prudishness or poor self-image and our feelings toward our partner, along with so many other things going on in our minds, affect our sex lives more than anything else. If we learn to be comfortable with ourselves, we are more likely to find and be able to give sexual pleasure. That may sound pollyannish, but it's hard to deny. Sex comes with so much emotional baggage that sometimes it's difficult to just relax and enjoy it regardless of what form *it* takes. Of all the obstacles to a happy sex life that can be thrown in senior's paths, couples being mad at one another about something may be the most common. Our time here isn't getting longer, so do something about that. Sex is a great gift, one that multiplies as it is shared instead of being used up.

A healthy body and affection and respect for one's partner are the greatest aphrodisiacs.

We've always had sex, but my husband is the "on, off, roll over and go to sleep" type. That really isn't something to look forward to for me so much anymore. I would like to try receiving oral sex from him, but he determined he doesn't care for that decades ago. Since he retired, he doesn't stay clean shaven, either, and I know that would be irritating even if we did it. -Female

I like the way sex columnist Michael Castleman put it in his September 30, 2009, article in *Psychology Today*: Fantasies During Sex: Welcome Them. "Sex is mutual meditation," he wrote. While partnered sex is the ultimate shared activity, what's going on in each participant's mind is still individual and private, no matter how cooperative the act. While it sounds nice to empty your mind and concentrate on nothing but your partner during sex, it's unlikely without disciplined meditative practice. From our youth, sex and fantasy are profoundly intertwined. Don't feel guilty about your fantasies. If they enhance your experience, embrace them back. It isn't being unfaithful to have thoughts about someone else, or some other situation or scenario, during sex. And, if your fantasies contain elements that can be incorporated into your sex life, be open enough to share them with your partner. Role playing? Saying things one wouldn't normally say? Long had a thing for vegetables or rubber chickens, or, just once, you would like to whisper *Laurie Partridge* or *Bobby Goldsboro* (or heck, Laurie Partridge *and* Bobby Goldsboro for that matter. I don't judge) at a strategic moment? Do you visualize yourself as Brad and your partner as Angelina, or vice versa in a movie scene (okay, I know they aren't a couple anymore)? Great. Your partner may not mind, or possibly even be intrigued. You will never know unless you ask. If it helps the two of you have fun together and keeps things moving, how can it be a bad thing?

It's nothing big, but I am embarrassed by it. When my husband and I make love, I say things in my mind I would never say out loud. I won't be specific, but things like I'm going to do something to your something, and you do something to me. You can probably figure it out. But he would die if I said anything like that out loud. We're church people. -Female

That's why getting over yourselves and your embarrassment and beginning to communicate openly about sex is what makes or breaks us. Too many of us who first began thinking about sex during the Age of Aquarius and who hitchhiked to Woodstock (I was only ten years old and was living in West Virginia, by the way, so it was out of the question for me) have inexplicably become our prudish, noncommunicative Greatest Generation grandparents when it comes to sex.

You know, those grandparents who had 16 children.

THE QUEST FOR INTIMACY vs. SEX

I have been divorced from an abusive husband for years and not been interested in dating any more men. It really surprised me when I started having physical attraction feelings for a close friend. We love being together and are very intimate emotionally. She's never been married. We moved in together and are very happy. I really don't see myself as being homosexual, but I just love her, and I know she loves me. We have a good life together, and we are physically intimate. Now some family members have nothing to do with us, even though from the outside we could just be two older single ladies living together to share expenses. But we're happy and it's none of their business. -Female

Truer words were never spoken, Female.

We were married for more than fifty years, and everything was fine, I guess. I have never, ever admitted it to anyone, but my whole life, when pleasuring myself, I fantasized about my very first sexual experience back when I was a teenager. And it wasn't with a girl. -Male

Accepting that one's sexuality may include shades of gray is probably easier for today's younger people than it was for Baby Boomers. It's also easier to find help sorting through and figuring out how to deal with long-buried emotions. Truth is a beast to tame, and honesty about oneself can be the most dangerous species of it. But once subdued, it can offer greater loyalty, contentment, and protection than any other.

For most of us most of the time, there is no complete separation between emotionally intimate relationships and sex, making both so much more complicated. "Cruise" and casual anonymous sex culture have become much easier and more acceptable by internet apps. Unfortunately, as ease of finding someone to have sex with increases, we are amid an emotional and social attachment crisis across the generations. Whether or not one leads to the other is still an important question, one uniquely individual and personal. Though I cannot point to a controlled study as evidence, my belief is that cultivation of both emotional and sexual intimacy, with professional assistance if needed, is at once extremely difficult and immensely satisfying. Being able to have both requires hard work and constant attention, despite our movie-inspired visions to the contrary. These days, it might even seem to require an abundance of luck and perhaps even Divine intervention, and, above all, flexibility, compromise, forgiveness, and being less self-centered just at a time of life when the default seems to become more so.   Homily over.

We're winding down, and it's time for some final sexy reflections.

THINK ABOUT IT: It's sex, sex, sex wherever you look, but not for us seniors, at least not in popular perception. Look at these statements:

1. Teenage boy masturbating, using a sex toy
2. 30-something woman masturbating, using a sex toy
3. Senior citizen in a nursing home masturbating, using a sex toy

You know very well the difference in the reactions those statements would bring, even among ourselves.

1. Heh! It's natural and expected. Just stay away from the pie. That's for dessert!
2. In the City, after buying outrageously expensive shoes? Hilarious! You go, girlfriend!
3. Ewwww, nasty. They shouldn't allow that.

Tell me I'm wrong? That senior citizen spent three years in Vietnam, worked as a truck driver for forty years, and he and his wife raised three kids, one of whom became a minister. Or, that senior citizen was the first of her family to go to college, was an underpaid elementary school teacher buying classroom supplies with her own meager salary for half a century, and she still longs for the feeling of her late husband beside her.

Perhaps either or both have dementia and, in their minds, are imagining a young lover from a lifetime ago. Maybe they're just old people bringing themselves a bit of pleasure in an otherwise drab existence. (While the latter scenario is the least romantic, it happens to be my favorite.) It's their right. No matter how much you pretend or wish otherwise, we are sexual beings, and will continue to be until our last breaths.

We deserve better. I don't care if we're partnered or single or living independently or in assisted living or in a nursing home, we deserve better. But it's not going to happen unless we make it. Senior citizens, even those no longer living independently, should not be deprived of the basic human right to have private solo or partnered sex if they willingly desire and are capable of consent. Because of embarrassment and taboos and elder discrimination, though, that may be the one paragraph that keeps this book out of libraries in some states. *He advocates people in nursing homes be given the privacy and resources to have sex and/or masturbate!!!*

I have always wanted to join the pantheon of banned book authors. It's good company.

Think what you want, but around me keep your disrespectful-to-our-elders *"Ewww"* to yourself. It's bad enough when popular culture dismisses seniors' sexual feelings as being inappropriate and gross, but it's even worse when we do it to ourselves. The guilt and self-loathing over sex that society thrusted upon us were unwarranted and unhealthy back in adolescence and remain so today.

While there are exceptions, it's plain our culture places more emphasis on sexuality among those younger than you and me. But the title of one article, sums it up: *What Keeps Passion Alive? Sexual Satisfaction Is Associated With Sexual Communication, Mood Setting, Sexual Variety, Oral Sex, Orgasm, and Sex Frequency in a National U. S. Study.* (22)

There you go. A checklist. Time's a-wastin'. It matters to you as a human being, regardless of your age, physical condition, or relationship status.

While most of the references and scenarios have alluded to heterosexual relationships, everything applies to whatever type of love you seek or find. There are instances of people who have lived their lives, sometimes quite happily, in heterosexual relationships, but find the freedom in later years to expand their circle of experiences. Be who you are and do what makes you happy. It's your business, your life, your happiness. Don't give up sex without a fight because it hasn't given up on *you*, no matter what society would have us believe.

THE TAKEAWAY

Muscles atrophy unless exercised, and your sex parts are muscles. However you can, with a partner or solo, orgasmic or simply pleasurable and relaxing, enjoy sex to the best of your ability. Always be respectful to both yourself and others, but also be open to trying new things, get over your old embarrassment and thoughts of loss and inadequacy, and simply feel pleasure. You will be a healthier, happier, more pleasant, and all-round better person for it.

Don't give up something good because it's not perfect, or "like it used to be." You're probably seeing the past through rose-colored glasses anyway. The most effective aphrodisiacs and sexual performance boosters are good overall health, confidence, mindfulness, and genuine affection for your sex partner (even if it's only yourself).

Openly and honestly communicate with your partner and your doctor. Make sure sex is part of medical and mental health conversations. Things don't have to be horrible for you to seek help making them better.

Do it for yourself.

And, when desired, *by* yourself.

Do it for your partner if you have one.

Do it for those who must be around you.

If it helps, hang a flag in your bedroom and do it for Old Glory. It doesn't really matter.

Just…you know.

What if I was wrong at the beginning of this chapter? Good sex is sex you're *having*, not remembering. So maybe it really is the *best sex ever* after all.

2 TALK THE WALK

You're going to die, and it will probably be sooner than it has been. But there are things you can do to make the time you have left better.

One of those things you can do is walk. A lot. You may go to the gym or the pool or get in and out of a golf cart 40 times or play pickle ball (dang, that thing took off, didn't it?) every Tuesday, and that's all great. Good for you! All movement is good. Like Nancy Sinatra's boots, though, human beings have evolved to walk, and that's just what you should do. Walking is more than just another of the many things that are good for you, like plenty of fiber and sex. Failure to walk is nothing short of dangerous.

The science is undeniable. Being sedentary puts you at risk of obesity, insomnia, osteoporosis, arthritis, balance disorders, hypertension, high cholesterol, Type 2 diabetes, stroke, heart disease, reduced lung function, and even cancer (especially breast, uterine, and colon), urinary tract problems, depression, and reduced overall cognitive ability. You may be twice as likely to develop Alzheimer's disease and other forms of dementia.

Yes, these harms can be mitigated with other forms of exercise, but nothing is safer, simpler, or more physically essential than putting one foot in front of the other. Up until very recently (only about 12,000 years ago in a 2-million-year evolution) in even the most "advanced" societies, walking was simply what Homo sapiens did, all the time, as hunter-gatherers.

Once again like sex, it is truly a "use it or lose it" proposition, a potential spiral toward losing independence. If walking becomes difficult and you walk less, walking becomes even more difficult and you even walk less, making it still more difficult, in a vicious cycle. Once someone loses mobility, it is harder to be self-sufficient and live on one's own without assistance. Being immobile may expose you to fewer stimuli, affecting motivation, memory, and overall mental acuity.

How stiff are you after sitting for a while? It's probably a given at our age. Getting out of the car after a long drive these days makes me think of my father, because I make the same groaning noise he did while doing it. One reason is that most of our joint cartilage has little direct blood supply, and it gets nutrition and lubrication primarily from the synovial fluid that gets squished around by the movement as we walk. Get out of breath? Start slow and build yourself up. You will notice a difference in less time than you think.

The Arthritis Foundation reports that people in their fifties and sixties are more than a third less likely to die in the next eight years if they exercise regularly. How's that for incentive? It's free. It can be done alone or with someone else. It can be done safely, you feel better afterwards, and you can suffer both mental and physical consequences without it. (Didn't we say something similar in Chapter 1?)

How to begin?

1. Assess your current walking regime and abilities. Be honest. Is there anywhere you walk where you feel uncomfortable or unsafe, even in your own home? If so, what could be done to make it more secure? How do you feel during and after? One way to objectively measure how much you walk is by using one of those irritating little digital step and distance counters. I have seen them sold for around $15. If you don't like that price tag, your phone will probably even do it for free. Of course, there's an app (in fact, many different to

choose from) for that! Tell your doctor what you are planning to do and see if she has any advice or cautions. Start where you are. If walking to the post box is all you do now, it's a beginning on which you can build. Every single step is beneficial to you. If it's only 50 today, it can be 55 tomorrow.

2. Buy a good pair of walking shoes and socks. There aren't a lot of things I suggest you spend money on, but don't scrimp on these. Instead of surfing on your phone for them while watching Seinfeld reruns (I have seen a total of one episode of it, by the way, and that was enough for me), go to an actual athletic shoe store and have someone who knows what she or he is doing help fit you. They aren't cheap, but it's a much better investment in your future than many other things on which you spend your money. As for your clothing, just wear what's comfortable, won't chafe, and gives you adequate UV ray protection. Melanoma isn't one of the bad things walking helps prevent! Wear the shoes and socks around for several days before increasing your walking, to break them in and make sure the fit is right. As your walking time increases, you may also need a comfortable-to-carry water bottle.

3. Walk where you already walk, just further or more times. If that becomes boring, expand your route and incorporate new ones to rotate into your routine. Go to almost any mall and you will see senior citizens purposely walking instead of shopping. In fact, you may at some point have said, "Look at them in their velour sweatsuits. That will never be me!" Well, LET IT BE YOU, while there are still a few malls left. Just beware walking past Cinnabon if you are weak-willed. If your outdoor route has potholes, cracked sidewalks, street crossings without walk signals, unrestrained dogs, or other potential hazards, scout out another. You need a safe, comfortable route so you can concentrate less on the pavement and more on the world.

4. In your everyday life, stop trying to save steps. I see folks my age burning fossil fuel driving up and down in parking lots until a closer space comes open, then see them immerge

from their vehicle looking like a little walk would probably have done them a world of good. That may sound judgmental, and I don't know their whole physical condition story, but it's often true. Many people in my small neighborhood have golf carts and I detect an inverse relationship between "using a golf cart" and "*should be* using a golf cart instead of walking.*" Buildings with elevators also have stairs. They get lonely. Reach out.

5. If you don't have an interested significant other, find a partner (That Chapter 1 advice keeps cropping up, doesn't it?). Casually ask neighbors. There may be people you already know who are walking. If you regularly encounter some, there's nothing wrong with asking to join them. It won't take more than half a mile for them to determine you aren't an ax murderer if, indeed, you are not one. Many communities, parks, gyms, and even malls have free walking programs, the latter hoping you eventually *do* give in to Cinnabon.

6. If you need a cane or wheeled walker, use one. "Oh, I don't like to hold other people up," is just an excuse for laziness and vanity. People can go around you and may benefit from a lesson in patience, because their day is coming.

7. Don't set a pace or distance that is painful. If it isn't enjoyable, you can talk yourself out of doing it. That little watch thingy or app will record your distance and pace. After a while, try 10% longer/faster. Stick with that until you are feeling good doing it, then try for another increase. You can also choose a segment of your walk to increase your pace, then slow back down. Over time, lengthen these faster distances. To pass the time more enjoyably, many people listen to music or podcasts on headsets. That's fine, but remember that you do need to be able to react to your surroundings. Headsetted (is that a word?) walkers may not hear bicycle bells and other warning sounds. Having a companion and chatting along the way is, I think, better because it also strengthens social connections and talking while walking may add to the lung capacity benefit.

8. Stretch before and after. This doesn't need to be elaborate. Just stretch, slowly and without jerking anything. Try tightening your belly muscles periodically as you walk, holding them in until it becomes uncomfortable, then relaxing for a time before you flex again.

All that is intuitive and do-able, tomorrow if not today. In addition, weight training is also necessary to keep from losing muscle mass as we age. Don't neglect it.

MENTAL, EMOTIONAL, SOCIAL, AND SPIRITUAL INPACT: A WALKING STORY

Walking is important to me. It is just about the only kind of exercise I enjoy that isn't addressed in Chapter 1. Beyond the health benefits, it can have great mental, emotional, social, and even spiritual impact as well, and I have a story to share. Some time ago, I was feeling a bit rudderless. I had retired from the federal court at age 51 a few years earlier, remarried, and moved 300 miles away from my hometown. I thought I would go back into the workforce for a few more years to feel productive, be part of something important, meet new people, and make a few bucks. I knew I wouldn't match my court salary, but that was okay. My wife Sandy, younger than me and an RN, was still working full time. Let's see…MA+45, management and teaching experience, etc. Should be easy to find something acceptable, right?

Crickets, as they say.

I needed purpose. That old soap opera opening with the big hourglass began to haunt me. The thing that had always helped clear my head best has been walking. My unscientific theory is that, in addition to increasing blood flow to the brain, it comes so naturally to us that it doesn't take up much of that organ's capacity, allowing us to work out problems in a program running in the background, so to speak. And, even while walking a familiar route, it's easy to see something along the way that causes you to think about some related thing that can trigger ideas.

Sand running out…An event that I won't go into occurred that pushed me out of the "someday I would like to" phase into actual planning. I had visited Scotland before and loved it. Walking there would be fun. That kind of trip did not interest my wife, so I began making tentative plans to go alone. Just in case, I put out the call on my Facebook page to see if any of my acquaintances wanted to join me but had little hope anyone would. I will always be profoundly grateful that I was wrong.

This book is dedicated to the memory of W. Mark Deskins, with whom I graduated from high school in 1977. We had lost contact for decades but reconnected not long before I retired. Mark was an engineer and an upper-level manager with the Department of the Navy. He loved to travel, had the time and resources, and, in his own words, "needed a good walk." He recruited his son Josh, also with the Department of the Navy and an engineer, to join us. I had not met Josh before. Soon Tammy, one of my New England cousins about a decade younger than me, and her husband Roland signed on as well. I am not sure they all understood the depth of my OCD when they agreed to leave all the planning up to me. Not even one of us knew all the others. When we all met up in the Reykjavik, Iceland airport for the last leg of the journey to Edinburgh and made our introductions, I felt like Gandalf assembling a fellowship of...something.

After an evening together in Edinburgh, our diverse band walked straight down the Royal Mile to pick up the last section (or first, depending on your direction) of the John Muir Way, a trail that cuts across the country from Glasgow to Dunbar, the naturalist's hometown on the North Sea coast.

The trail is described as "fairly well marked," with the term "fairly" being as broad as Scottish brogue itself.

It was one of the best experiences of my life. I began walking my own neighborhood as soon as our plans were set, and I became healthier and happier as a result. I learned many things about my surroundings and interacted with people. When we got to Scotland, the simple act of walking bound us together in a unique way. For each of us, the memories and friendships forged while dodging thistles and scowling at rainclouds and drinking dark, bitter beer in the evenings while on a walk will follow us to the grave. I came back with wee toe blisters and more direction in my life. We all did.

Just a couple of years later, during a particularly demanding and challenging time at work, Mark called me and said, "I need to walk again. How about Ireland?' And so we did, with a whole new set of characters other than Mark and me. The Fellowship of the Trail, Irish Edition included Mark's other son Matthew, Quaye (a young neighbor of mine), Godfrey (a retired dentist friend of Mark's originally from the Caribbean), Dee (a lawyer friend with whom I attended college) and Dee's husband Brian, a retired machinist. It was just as edifying, head-clearing, relationship-building and everything else as the Scottish walk. It had great mental, emotional, social, and even spiritual impact for us all.

I talked with both Mark and Dee about this writing project and asked them to write a blurb about the impact of our walks together.

Ladies first.

Five years ago, when approaching the age of 60, I had the chance to join a walking tour of the Kerry Way in Ireland. Having never been to Ireland, I jumped at the chance. It turned out to be one of the best and most memorable travel experiences of my life! For several days, we traversed the Irish countryside, climbing over numerous "stiles" and passing farmhouses, herds of sheep, and beautiful shorelines. The long hours of hiking over some rough terrain in rainy weather sometimes pushed me to the limit. Each evening, however, a quaint new town, delightful Irish pub, and bed & breakfast awaited us! So glad I decided to walk the Kerry Way and explore Ireland this way! I thoroughly enjoyed the scenery, the history, and most of all the fellowship with old friends and new! When is our next trip? - Dee

As I have gotten older, I recognized that I can do nothing significant except help the people around me. Whether it is just spending time with people, catching up with old friends, or doing a "chore" for someone, it is important to connect with others. I hadn't seen Danny for almost 30 years until we reconnected at our high school reunion. We seemed to pick up where we left off and continued to communicate through email and Facebook. His post on Facebook caught my attention. Go visit Scotland and take a break. I was ready to put some of the recent life events (9/11, Navy Yard shooting, parents' death) behind me and a vacation was what I needed. I thought. "Maybe I'll be able to use some of my Marriott points," but that was not to happen. Instead, it set the stage for another life journey. - Mark

You don't have to go to Scotland or Ireland or anywhere else but outside your own door to walk, and there is most likely someone out there to share the journey with you.

THE TAKEAWAY

Human beings are meant to walk. There is no simpler, cheaper, safer way to improve your health than getting out of your chair. It doesn't matter how little you can do at first. Simply walk. The positive effects are not only physical, but **flow over into every aspect of our lives.**

Social isolation is bad for you, both physically and mentally. Walking with someone else is cheap, easy, doesn't require much planning or division of duties, and walking conversations and relationships can be either as superficial or intimate as you like. Walking as a communal activity can help mitigate isolation as a serious mental and physical health risk factor. Get up and do it.

3 STILL FLYING HIGH

You're going to die, and it will probably be sooner than it has been. But there are things you can do to make the time you have left better.

Honesty in self-evaluation is an uncomfortable thing when it comes to drinking.

I have a little off-grid cabin in the mountains. It's on almost five beautiful rolling acres, uses a cistern as a water source, has comfortable beds, lots of books, solar lightning, a composting toilet (why my wife doesn't accompany me there) and I love sitting out by the fire pit at night under the canopy of stars, listening to music. My kind of music. While doing this, alone with my thoughts and enjoying the night sky and the coolness of the country setting and the best music ever recorded, I have drinks.

When I was young, I thought we were on a slow but steady trajectory towards freedom and equality. I lived in Green Fields, Had a Hammer, didn't Give a Damn About a Greenback Dollar, thought we would Overcome, knew Which Side I Was On, Where the Flowers Had Gone, where to Turn Turn Turn, and exactly what War was Good For. Now look at us. Good Gawd, Y'all. So I sit there and listen and drink and time stands still and I wake up the next morning not really remembering much of it. -Male

I feel ya, man. Drinking is so often situational and compensates for boredom. My wife worked nightshift in the Surgical ICU for years. On winter evenings, I would watch television with "a couple glasses" of wine. Two factors often ruled my evenings. 1. You can find many of the old *Smothers Brothers Comedy Hour, Hullabaloo, Hootenanny, American Bandstand, Ed Sullivan* (where was the chemistry between the taciturn Sullivan and Topo Gigio, anyhow? What was the nature of their relationship? It remains a mystery to me), and *Shindig!* shows on YouTube, and 2. an opened bottle of wine quickly goes flat in the refrigerator. Right?

I live in a convenient neighborhood, and in less than ten minutes can walk to the movie theater and bookstore. I can also be at Gordon Biersch, Tupelo Honey, the Brass Tap, Tidal Creek Brew House, King Street Grill, or Travinias, all of which have happy hours. My wife's dog, when she was with us, was even welcome at the patio bars and was quite a regular. A celebrity, even! After a couple beers, the little Cavalier King Charles Spaniel wanted to swish her wispy tail down to the lake and take on a couple of the resident Canada geese, until she came within a dozen feet of them. Then she wanted carried.

Whenever friends say, "Let's get together!" I know what we gather to do will most likely include food (even if it's just snacks) and something to wash it down.

I go to the book club meeting and a few members mention something about the book, but mainly we drink wine. Our monthly Ladies Business Luncheon is the same way. If we go to the pool, we pack a cooler of hard seltzer. Meeting a friend for dinner means taking an Uber back home. Having a social life is important and I enjoy it, but every activity is centered around eating and, mainly, drinking. -Female

You get the picture. So many activities, whether social or solitary, include alcohol. We can justify it easily enough. I worked hard all those years, now I really enjoy sitting around that fire pit, listening to music, having a few. Yep, this is just what I looked forward to all those years. I deserve it. And it could be leading to illness or even a premature death.

Like most people, I have drunk alcohol to some degree since adolescence, beginning back when the legal drinking age was 18 but my aforementioned late friend Mark and I used my Dad's expired driver's license to buy beer at 17. (How on earth did they let us get by with that? Did I *look* like I was born the year the Great Depression hit?) In college (especially as an undergraduate at Marshall University) and on rare occasions afterward, I *may have* overindulged a bit. But afterwards, while busy being the parent of two daughters and having a career, it was easier to let moderation rule. Usually. Almost always. Or at least frequently.

Then came retirement. I have lots of time. I still rise early though I seldom need to do so. Every day is a holiday, and holidays are made for celebration, even if it's a party of one.

I'm not alone. The U. S. Department of Health and Human Services (DHHS) SAMHSA (Substance Abuse and Mental Health Services Administration) spends substantial resources on tracking these things, because they are major public health concerns. Its 2021 *National Survey on Drug Use and Health* is as scientific and comprehensive as we can get. It found that alcohol use among older adults is increasingly problematic, with approximately 20% of adults aged 60-65 self-reporting binge drinking. That's one in five people my age *admitting* it.

Like most other functions, our ability to process alcohol slows down as we age, and we may suffer the effects of it more quickly than we once did, putting us at higher risk of just about anything negative that can happen, whether it be unintentional injury or gradual harm to our bodies. Heavy drinking can exacerbate diabetes, hypertension, heart failure, liver disease, kidney disease, osteoporosis, memory difficulty, mood disorders, sexual dysfunction, you name it. Since elders are more likely to take medication, interactions with aspirin, acetaminophen, cold and allergy medicine, cough syrup, sleeping pills, pain medication, anxiety or depression medicines and a host of other drugs, both prescription and over the counter, are more common.

Alcohol is believed to be a factor in almost a third of suicides and fatal car crashes, 40% or fatal burn injuries, half of fatal drownings and homicides, and 65% of fatal falls.

The current DHHS guidelines state that older adults can certainly abstain from alcohol altogether, but, if they do drink, should consume no more than two drinks a day for men and one for women. And certain adults should refrain altogether.

What is a drink? One 12-ounce serving of regular beer, ale, or hard seltzer, one 8-ounce bottle of malt liquor, one 5-ounce glass of wine, or one 1.5-ounce measure of 80-proof liquor, either as a shot or mixed in a cocktail.

That is important information. You can easily tell yourself you are having just two glasses of wine, but a half bottle will fit in my wine glass, and one bottle is more than five servings. A single cocktail accepted from my friend nicknamed "Don't Let Kevin Pour," for example, can easily put one way over the limit.

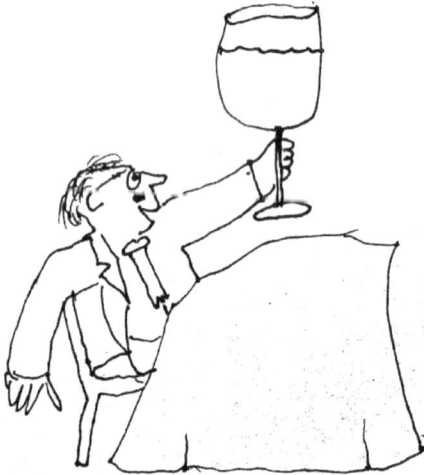

"So I sez to Doc, 'Nope, just one glass a day for me, Doc,' I sez."

Hey, I thought a glass of wine or two is beneficial, especially to older folks? There are so many mixed results. The Mayo Clinic, relying on studies by C. C. Tangney and K. J. and others, concludes that, while more research is needed, it appears those who drink moderate amounts of alcohol (including but not limited to red wine) seem to have a lower risk of heart disease. Alcohol may raise the HDL "good cholesterol" levels, reduce the formation of blood clots, help prevent artery damage caused by LDL "bad cholesterol," and be protective of the cells that line the blood vessels. (23)

I'm pretty sure drinking is good for our health. Every evening my husband and I have cocktails out on the patio. After having cocktails, we don't drive anywhere, meaning we don't cruise the Dairy Queen drive through for ice cream! See? Healthy! - Female

Nice try. The potential protective effects, according to the American Heart Association and National Heart, Lung, and Blood Institute, aren't significant enough to recommend you start drinking, even in moderation, if you aren't already doing so. The Mayo Clinic's recommendation mirrors the DHHS for younger people at up to two drinks a day for men up to age 65 and one drink a day for women of all ages, but *only one drink a day for men older than 65*.

Dang. One drink. That's supposed to get you through *The Ed Sullivan Show* episode with The Mamas and the Papas where John Phillips was so obviously stoned?

I don't drink every day. Sometimes I will go a whole week without drinking at all. But when I do, it's easy to tell myself it's a reward for having been good all week and end up drinking way too much. If my wife has a drink, she wants me to have one with her so she's not drinking alone, naturally. We put out some cheese and nuts and watch TV and before you know it, I've had six drinks in the course of the evening. But it only happens occasionally, so I'm not sure it's really a problem. I mean, if I were an alcoholic, I wouldn't go a week without drinking at all and not even think about it, would I?" -Male

No, you can't safely "save up" your daily alcohol consumption to be downed all in one sitting. Darn.

There is sometimes confusion between the terms alcoholic, heavy drinking, and binge drinking. According to the National Institute of Health's National Institute on Alcohol Abuse and Alcoholism, binge drinking is a pattern of drinking alcohol that brings the blood alcohol concentration (BAC) to 0.08 or more. How much alcohol that takes depends on your size, age, etc. It's on the rise for us seniors. Even one episode of binge drinking cam compromise function of the immune system and lead to acute pancreatitis. Add that to the single binge-increased risk of falls, car crashes, and all kinds of *"Hey, guys, watch this"* incidences during old buddy golf trips, and it's a major senior health concern. It's common for us to have that one circumstance, that one place, that one acquaintance that triggers us to overindulge.

Do you really want your falling into a drunken slumber to be what people remember most about your granddaughter's bat mitzvah afterparty, even if you are the one footing the bar bill?

And just what is a "problem drinker?" If your drinking is negatively affecting your mental or physical health or your relationships, it is a problem, regardless of whether you meet the somewhat subjective criteria of being an alcoholic.

Do you often drink more than you intended? Is there ever really such a thing as an unfinished bottle of wine in your refrigerator?

Do you think about wanting a drink when things aren't going well, you're stressed, or bored? Is alcohol part of your default coping strategy?

Do you ever have regrets or guilt about how much you drink, or hide how much you are drinking from others? Do you sometimes not remember what you watched on television while you were drinking, or wake up to find you had made a post on social media (Boy, those can be fun) or an online purchase you don't remember?

Does being alone (and unmonitored) change the amount you drink?

Do you drink your drinks down relatively fast?

Do you ever drive after having consumed alcohol? (Attention residents of Myrtle Beach, South Carolina: Yes, that includes a GOLF CART or BOAT!)

Do you view drinking as your "reward," something you "deserve" for having worked hard all those years?

The results of a study referenced by Harvard Medical School on September 24, 2021, found Alcohol Use Disorder among people over 65 increased a full 107% between 2001 and 2013. The University of Michigan's Healthy Aging poll, cited in the same article, found that 20% of the older respondents drank alcohol four or more times a week, 27% had six or more drinks on at least one occasion in the past year, and 7% reported alcohol-related blackouts. That's huge.

The first step (and I am determined to take my own advice here) is to be honest with yourself *and your doctor* about how much you drink. It is easy to drastically underestimate it. Use a measure to determine if that "single glass of wine" really is just one serving. If you don't drink (which is a perfectly acceptable option, even if you have used alcohol all your life. Your body and mind and medications change over time, and so can your preferences about drinking, and that's fine) it's nobody's business but your own. If your actual consumption is within the guidelines and doesn't cause any other issues (due to meds, etc.), that's a good sign. But, after an honest evaluation, you find you are drinking too much, what do you do?

Harvard Medical School (24) offers this excellent list of suggestions, without beating us on the heads with a fire and brimstone admonition to become teetotalers (with a few of my own comments thrown in):

Put it in writing. Making a list of the reasons to curtail your drinking — such as feeling healthier, sleeping better, or improving your relationships — can motivate you.

Set a drinking goal (Boy, does that have a different meaning now than it did as a college freshman!). Set a limit on how much you will drink, and even share it with your significant other. You should keep your drinking below those pesky recommended guidelines. Repeat: no more than one standard drink per day for women and for men ages 65 and older, and no more than two standard drinks per day for men under 65. Those limits may be too high for people who have certain medical conditions or for some other older adults. Your doctor can help you determine what's right for you.

Keep an honest diary of your drinking. For three to four weeks, keep track of every time you have a drink. Include information about what and how much you drank as well as where you were. Compare this to your goal. If you're having trouble sticking to your goal, discuss it with your doctor or another health professional.

Don't keep much alcohol in your house. Having no alcohol at home can help limit your overall drinking, because there may not be enough time to get to the liquor store and back before the *PBS Newshour* comes on.

Drink slowly. Sip your drink. Drink soda, water, or juice after having an alcoholic beverage. Never drink on an empty stomach. My personal strategy that has served me well since the Carter administration: drink as much water as you do alcoholic beverage at the same sitting. If I am out with someone and have two beers at a pub, my goal is to also have drunk two glasses of water. The extra hydration is good for you. It increases time between drinks, fills you up, and may even help prevent hangovers. Just know where the bathrooms are, both in the pub and along the way home.

Choose alcohol-free days. Decide not to drink a day or two each week. You may want to abstain for a week or a month to see how you feel physically and emotionally without alcohol in your life. Taking a break from alcohol can be a good way to start drinking less overall. I have embraced Dry January. It gives the body a good rest from alcohol after the holidays and may give you some insight as to just how big a role alcohol plays in your life. I used to do the same for Lent as well. Join with others for mutual support and it shouldn't be difficult. Plus, assuring yourself you have the willpower to complete Dry January may counteract that sense of failure you experienced attempting No Nut November, but that's a Chapter 1 subject.

Watch for peer pressure. Practice ways to say *no* politely. You do not have to drink just because others are, and you shouldn't feel obligated to accept any drink you're offered. Stay away from people who encourage you to drink. Ask for an old-fashioned glass filled with your choice of brown or clear pop (soda to you non-Appalachians) with a lime wedge and cherry, and only the bartender will know the difference, until your friends wonder why you haven't done your signature Bob Dylan impression all evening.

Keep busy. Take a walk, play sports, go out to eat, or catch a movie. When you're at home, pick up a new interest or revisit an old one. Painting, reading, board and card games, playing a musical instrument, woodworking — these and other activities are great alternatives to drinking. If those don't grab your interest, re-read Chapter 1.

Ask for support. Cutting down on your drinking may not always be easy. Let friends and family members know that you need their support. Your doctor, counselor, or therapist may also be able to offer help.

Guard against temptation. Steer clear of people and places that make you want to drink. If you associate drinking with certain events, such as holidays or vacations, develop a plan for managing them in advance. Monitor your feelings. When you're worried, lonely, or angry, you may be tempted to reach for a drink. Try to cultivate new, healthy ways to cope with stress. Be persistent. Most people who successfully cut down or stop drinking altogether do so only after several attempts. You'll probably have setbacks, but don't let them keep you from reaching your long-term goal. There's no real endpoint, as the process usually requires ongoing effort.

It's counterintuitive to give up something you enjoy, especially when you may have more time to do it and see that big Hourglass of Life's sand running out. You may enjoy drinking, and feel that, since you have worked hard throughout your life, you deserve to do what you enjoy. You've waited all these years to eat, drink, and be merry without looking at the clock!

Good for you. But, reaching for too much gusto can make that sand run faster and more painfully. For most seniors, there is a way to enjoy things without inflicting harm on ourselves and our loved ones. Don't be embarrassed to reach out for help finding it. A place to start may be the Substance Abuse and Mental Health Services Administration's (a division of the U. S. Department of Health and Human Services) free 24/7, 356-days-a-year, free and confidential helpline. The number is 1-800-662-HELP (4357). That resource can apply to all topics in this chapter.

STILL SMOKIN'

You know what I'm talking about.

Marijuana (or, as it was affectionally called among the coalfield first-generation-going-to-college boys on the tenth floor of Twin Towers East at Marshall University in the 1970s, "squeebie," a vegetative matter to be "huffed," as in "Rocky was huffin' squeebie getting ready for the concert but then fell asleep and missed the whole thing") has never appealed to me. I smoked it a total of about a dozen times, all from 1977-79. The timing turned out to be good. When I filled out my questionnaire for an FBI background investigation prior to becoming a United States Probation Officer in 1990, the marijuana question specified "within the past 10 years." Clean living pays off, friends. (Full confession: a couple of years before the pandemic, "retired me" had an extended gig doing training programs for the federal court in Los Angeles. I was there for 18 days, including a long holiday weekend off. Since it is legal for recreational use in California, I briefly considered going to a dispensary and buying mild gummies or brownies and trying it once again, after 40+ years. But I was alone and a bit nervous about it and wanted to fully enjoy the La Brea Tar Pit experience during my time off, so I reconsidered)

Had I written this book a decade ago, I may have had a more judgmental attitude. "What!? Y'all still smokin' dope at your age? Grow up why don't ya, and pour me another Guinness" comes to mind. But all that has changed. In almost half the states, there are circumstances in which you can smoke marijuana legally, though you may still be breaking federal law. As the children of the 70s and 80s gained positions of power, cultural and legal norms began shifting.

Before we get to recreational use, let's talk about the medical side of it. In addition to potential pain and anxiety relief, improved sleep, and increased appetite, marijuana use can, according to some research, sometimes even improve cognitive functioning, probably because of those very things: pain control and improved sleep. This is according to a 2018 study primarily conducted by researchers at McLean Hospital in Belmont, Massachusetts. (25) It is also being studied for its potential use in the treatment of Parkinson's Disease.

The overall problem with determining the safety and effectiveness of marijuana in all its forms (smoking, edibles, THC or the less potently psychoactive CBD, etc.) is the lack of research. Unfortunately, the "War on Drugs" prevented adequate research on the possible benefits of marijuana and many other substances for decades, and the medical community is playing catch up. Some recent findings on senior marijuana use are noted in an article in *U. S. News and World Reports* (January 16, 2023) by Cara Murez cites statistics from the University of California, San Diego, the *Journal of the American Medical Association*, and the *Journal of the American Geriatrics Society*. Those sources are all prestigious medical heavy hitters. The research shows that older people who use marijuana, in whatever form, often do so to treat pain, sleep problems, anxiety, and depression.

It is also increasingly used to counteract some of the effects of chemo, and for cancer patients' pain and anxiety management. My father died of lung cancer at age 79, back before medical marijuana was available. His last six months were miserable, and I felt very sorry for him. He had no appetite and wasted away to around 90 pounds, always felt nauseated, and was scared. I remember thinking then, even as someone with very limited marijuana experience, that some of the effects commonly associated with marijuana could really benefit Dad. If there had been a legal way that didn't involve smoking (which his condition would have prevented) for him to feel less sick and anxious and maybe get a munchie attack before sleeping better, I would have been all for it.

There are repercussions. The number of seniors who wind up in the ER with adverse cannabis reactions increased well over 1,500% between 2005 and 2019. Why? Three factors: the drug is so much easier to obtain and less stigmatized now that it has been widely legalized or decriminalized, it can interact with other medications (particularly anti-seizure medications, and blood thinners) people are taking, and the marijuana available today is night-and-day different from that seniors may remember from their own adolescence, leading to considerable overdosing. Typical reactions include dizziness and falls, heart palpitations, panic attacks, confusion, anxiety, or worsening of underlying lung diseases, such as asthma or COPD. Inhaling smoke of any type is harmful to the lungs, and, like tobacco, marijuana smoke has been found to contain carcinogens.

I suspect, regardless of surveys and research studies, many seniors say they use marijuana medicinally, but really do so because they enjoy it.

That's nothing new. My paternal grandfather only took whiskey "medicinally," but was darned conscientious about not missing a dose. Many have never stopped using it from their hippie days and are in their seventh decade toking up. Remember that marijuana, in whatever form, can still impair your reflexes and decision making, just like alcohol. Driving, walking, and other activities that require coordination and judgement can be affected. Also remember that possession of marijuana is still a federal crime, everywhere in the country, and technically can be prosecuted even in state jurisdictions legalizing it. Walking down the street in Chicago or Manhattan or Philadelphia or Los Angeles any time day or night and drawing a deep breath will indicate how seldom that happens.

I live in a community with lots of retired folks, in a state with neither medicinal nor recreational marijuana legalization. When someone new moves in nearby, I find a way to drop into conversation that the robust smell of marijuana often present in the back alley is not coming from *my* garage. The culprit (or at least the one I know…there are probably others) is midway into his 80s. Yet another neighbor also older than me will openly share his recipe for a marijuana/DMSO tincture that he swears helps his back pain when used topically.

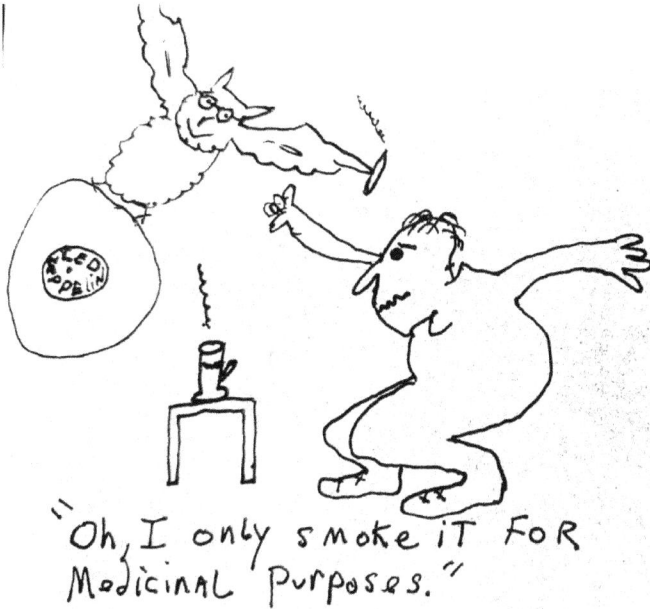

"Oh, I only smoke it for Medicinal Purposes."

Go to it, friends, if that's your thing. If it helps, it helps. But you'll find the Kuhns mixing Saturday morning mimosas on the front patio instead, and you're welcome to join us. Don't bring brownies. And don't drive while huffing squeebie.

OTHER VICES

Just like with marijuana, I must rely on science rather than personal experience when writing about tobacco and illegal narcotics, since I use neither. (Though, when I was young, I did have a brief affair with pipe smoking. I was the academic type and thought it might give me a distinguished look, like it did Robert Oppenheimer...who died of throat cancer. At age 62.) We will address legal narcotics separately, a bit later.

It doesn't matter how old you are, or for how many decades you have smoked, quitting now can improve your health, and you should do it. You are likely to live longer, breathe more easily, have more energy, lower your risk of cancer, heart disease, stroke, osteoporosis, blindness, diabetes, and lung disease. You will have better blood circulation, improved sense of taste and smell, and more money in your pocket. Nicotine is a highly addictive drug delivered in a manner that also injects carcinogens into your body and clogs your lungs. Other than addiction, there's no legitimate excuse for not quitting.

But if I quit smoking, I'll gain weight. My Dad smoked a pack a day and lived to be 94. If it's not hurt me by now, quitting isn't going to make a difference this late in the game. I don't really believe what they say about secondhand smoke; my wife doesn't get enough of it to hurt her!

Bull stuff. Go volunteer at your local hospice house and visit someone dying of lung cancer. Talk with someone who uses an Electrolarynx to communicate after having had a laryngectomy. Will quitting today guarantee that won't be your fate? No, but it will lessen the chances, even after lighting up for half a century or more.

According to the *Journal of the American Medical Association* (October 24, 2022), your odds aren't particularly good, and I won't lie to you about them. Although approximately 30% to 50% of smokers in the United States try to quit in any given year, only 7.5% succeed. Intervention is the key.

What to do: Talk to your doctor. If she or he doesn't seem enthusiastic about intervention or lacks faith in it working, find another one. Call the National Cancer Institute's Smoking Quitline at 877-448-7848. It's all too easy to be smug about another's vice when you don't share it, but time has painfully cured me of that. Good luck, and I mean that sincerely.

"HARD" DRUGS: While illicit drug use usually declines after young adulthood, nearly a million American adults 65+ live with this type of substance abuse disorder. (26) There needs to be additional study of illicit drug abuse during the golden years, but frankly, hard drug addicts are less likely to be around to reach "golden" status. If this is an issue for you at our stage of life, my saying "get help" is of little consequence. You have already tried. Please try again.

PRESCRIPTION NARCOTICS

There are older folks out there who would never even think of using illegal drugs, those who believe kids out there using "dope" are the downfall of our civilization, all while being perfectly legal drug addicts themselves. I have known more than one. Sadly, our society did just about everything possible to get American "housewives" addicted to drugs during the June Cleaver years: Now that the kids are at school all day and the husband either at work, out with the boys, or inattentive, Sally may understandably become depressed. And, of course, she wants to remain slim so Herb doesn't start noticing that petite young secretary at the office. Her doctor asks how she feels these days, and, if she's honest, she tells (almost always a) him about it. Listless. No energy.

Boy, does he have an easy answer for you, Sal! With the stroke of a pen, she is on her way to becoming an amphetamine addict. And when the effects of the addiction begin showing themselves ("Now I have trouble sleeping, doctor."), no problem! Here's a script for "sleeping pills" and one for "daytime tranquilizers," just in case. I love looking at the ads in vintage magazines (I really am such a fun guy!) and it is gobsmacking how many ads for amphetamines and barbiturates there are, specifically aimed at women. "Now she can cope…thanks to Butisol (sodium butabarbital), "daytime sedative" for everyday stress!" That ad is accompanied by an image of a happy young woman in a housedress playing with her children. Go online or to an antique store and look at them yourself.

The late 60s and 70s brought new names into the household, as more women entered the workforce. Valium and Quaaludes became grist for standup comics as well as for suburban medicine cabinets.

All those were for mood, sleep, etc. What about pain? It was the heyday of synthetic opioids, such as Propoxyphene, most common in those days under the trade names Darvon and Darvocet, both of which have now been banned by the Food and Drug Administration.

We are living amid a great opioid crisis, and chances are most people reading this have been touched by it in some way. According to the Centers for Disease Control, around 130 Americans die from opioid overdose *each day*. My home state of West Virginia has the highest opioid overdose death rate in the

United States. It is a state with an older population that mainly worked in hard physical labor professions such as coal mining, lumbering, or farming, low average income, and a shortage of economic opportunities. What it does have, though, are pharmacies, almost as plentiful as Dollar General stores.

Williamson, West Virginia is in the state's southeastern coalfields, on the Tug River bordering Kentucky. It is the heart of Hatfield and McCoy country, with just about everyone I met there being related to those two families. My first job out of college was as a social worker there for two years, and it was there I met my first wife. Through her, my daughters and grandchildren are both Hatfield and McCoy descendants. The town has about 3,000 residents. Between 2008 and 2015, drug wholesalers distributed more than *20.8 million* prescription painkillers, mainly hydrocodone and oxycodone, to just two pharmacies, four blocks apart.

You read that right. Total population 3,000, and 20.8 million pills. (27) There have been lawsuits, both civil and criminal, with drug companies and drug store chains agreeing to pay huge sums of money, and politicians gleefully accept it to run their states so they can thump their chests about balancing the budget and lowering taxes (mainly for rich people) while citizens young and old continue to slump over dead in their cars or in the Quickie Mart bathroom.

Forgive me for my rather subjective and personal diversion concerning my home state, but it's the truth, and they are my people. So there.

In the *Harvard Health Blog* article Is an Opioid Really the Best Medication for My Pain? (June 19, 2019), Drs. Salim Zerriny and David Boyce do an excellent job of providing information to answer the title question, and I relied on their work to help explain it.

You have pain. I have pain. We're getting old. You expect something different? But what *kind* of pain makes the difference on what to do about it, what to ask for, and what to accept, both as something to live with as uncomfortable but inevitable and tolerable, and as proposed treatment.

Many of us have been asked to describe our pain on a scale from one to ten and have trouble doing it. When considering pain medication, there are two primary factors:

Classification: *Nociceptive pain* is the most common form of pain, caused by some sort of stimulus, i.e., inflammatory, chemical, or physical. It causes your skin, muscles, joints, bones, or organs to send an Ouch! message to your brain via nerves. *Neuropathic pain* is caused by an injury to the nerve itself. It's often described with such terms as shooting, burning, stabbing, electric shock, tingling, numbness, pins and needles, that sort of thing. It can originate from diabetes, shingles, autoimmune disorders, stroke, or cancer. One of the strangest types of neuropathic pain is that in which an amputated appendage still "hurts." My father lost half his left hand in an industrial accident when he was sixteen years old and occasionally complained of those long-gone two fingers hurting him at night.

Time course: *Acute pain* lasts less than three to six months (sometimes much less) and goes away once the underlying source is resolved. Post op surgical pain or a broken bone will be acute. *Chronic pain* lasts longer and over time can change the way the brain perceives pain sensations. Arthritis, back injury, and degrading joints can cause chronic pain, as well as the much less defined fibromyalgia.

Figuring out exactly what type of pain you have can be difficult, and as we age, they can overlap considerably. They all hurt, and we don't want to hurt. But here is a very important thing to remember: Opioids are not generally recommended or even effective in treating neuropathic pain. If you are being prescribed them for that kind of discomfort, question it. "You're not a doctor," you rightfully say. No, I am not, and I am not dispensing medical advice. I am saying you should be knowledgeable and involved and question important things.

A short-term course of opioids, typically three to seven days, prescribed following an injury or surgical procedure, is usually quite safe. But look: A large 2017 study by the CDC referenced by Drs. Zerriny and Boyce indicates that, in first time opioid users, one in seven who received a refill or a second prescription *was still using opioids a year later*. The brain builds up tolerance, and the user needs the opiate to simply feel normal.

The 2018 *National Survey on Drug Use and Health*, conducted by the Substance Abuse and Mental Health Services Administration, revealed 1.3% of seniors polled reported misuse of opioids during the past year. Now, that's people *admitting* misuse. Few folks prescribed opiates for chronic pain are likely to call it that. Opiates are the second most reported substance of abuse by seniors (after alcohol) and, by one estimate, up to 11% of seniors abuse prescription drugs. (28)

That's a lot of people and is likely to include someone reading this right now.

Broken record time: if you have a long-term, ongoing prescription for an opiate, talk to your doctor. These aren't things that should be on autopilot. And if your doctor thinks they are, get a second opinion. The University of Michigan National Poll on Healthy Aging (July 2018) found that 29% of older adults had received an opioid prescription within the past two years, most commonly for arthritis-related pain, back pain, surgery, or injury. They also reported health care providers and pharmacists did not consistently discuss appropriate use. Half said they kept leftover opioids after they felt better "in case they might need them again."

Educate yourself. Don't fall into the name trap. I have heard, "Oh, I only take Tylenol for pain." Yeah, right. You are taking the maximum dose of Tylenol 4, which is acetaminophen combined with codeine, an opiate with addiction potential.

It's not just narcotics, of course. Benzodiazepines used to treat anxiety or insomnia, for example (brand names Valium, Xanax, Klonopin, Ativan, and others) can also become addictive. These drugs are generally understood to be best prescribed for short-term use, but sometimes patients remain on them for a lifetime. Inform yourself and ask about potential alternatives.

SO MANY DRUGS

The National Institute on Aging, in its August 24, 2021 publication *The Dangers of Polypharmacy and the Case for Deprescribing in Older Adults*, rings a warning bell about seniors being prescribed too many medications. It cites a CDC report indicating 83% of adults in their 60s and 70s used at least one prescription drug in the past month, and a third used five or more. That's a whole lot of prescription meds, and there is no such thing as a drug without some sort of side effect. Excessive or unnecessary medications can increase the risk of adverse effects, including falls, harmful drug interactions with or impeding the benefit from both other prescription and over-the-counter meds, and cognitive impairment.

This uncharted field of "de-prescribing" seems counterintuitive in our society. Watch television. Read magazines. People are clearly happier and do many more adventurous things by taking more and more prescription meds with names that border on nonsensical. "I used to worry about things all the time, but then I discovered Lifesbreezy." When we go to the doctor, we want her to do something about it, whatever that "it" happens to be. We expect to walk out with a prescription.

You have been with your doctor for years. You trust her and don't really want to question her judgement. How, then, do you complete a deep review of your medications?

-Make a complete and accurate list of what medications currently being taken, including over-the-counter meds you take on your own.

-Make sure you know the proper name of each drug and for what it is prescribed. Ask if there are any that may no longer be necessary, or dosages reduced.

-Discuss any new symptoms and ask if any of your drugs might be causing them.

-Consider potential harms from the medications. Ask questions like, "Can this drug affect my memory?" "Can this drug increase my risk of falling?" Then have a discussion with your doctor about whether these benefits and risks make sense, and if not, if there are alternative options.

-If your doctor seems reluctant or offended by your active questioning, get another opinion.

Sometimes, common sense and quality of life issues can butt heads with accepted medical protocol. For example: my father was diagnosed with high cholesterol for the first time in his life when he had fewer than six months to live. His doctor, following protocol I assume, prescribed a statin and told Dad to cut down on meat and to switch to skim milk.

The man had lung cancer and was clearly dying. We trashed the statin prescription, and skim milk, which he hated, never entered the house. If he had wanted bacon-wrapped foie gras washed down by a chocolate milkshake for breakfast every morning at that point, that's what I would have gotten for him.

THE TAKEAWAY

There may be fewer restraints on our alcohol and drug use after retirement because we have more time and fewer responsibilities. After the novelty wears off, we can become bored. From the outside, sitting by the pool or on the patio listening to music and having drinks may seem like "the life," and we can be dishonest with ourselves about the harm we are doing by seeing drinking as a privilege, an entitlement earned through all those years of hard work. Having fewer social connections can lead to almost every opportunity "getting together" with others being viewed as celebratory and alcohol worthy. Being honest with yourself about your drinking is both hard and important. Do it and keep doing it. Unless the honest answer is *no, I don't drink more than I should,* then do something about it. That might be something you can just map out and do completely on your own but seek and accept help if not. There are alternatives when you are bored or getting together with friends or celebrating. Find them.

Unless you have been a life-long marijuana smoker, there is probably no good reason to take up the habit unless you do so for some perceived positive health effect, and that would need to be quite substantial to outweigh the potential harm. As stigma and legal risk decline and alternative delivery methods (edibles, etc.) are available, more research is desperately needed, but politics often prevents it. In the meantime, every carnival barker will try to separate you from your money with miracle CBD elixirs. Use caution.

Opiate prescriptions are extremely common, even for types and degrees of pain for which there may be safer alternatives. Insist on them, and view opiates as short-term necessities only, unless and until the sand is truly about to run out.

Don't be surprised if your every complaint is met with a new prescription by your doctor. It may be far more common to add new prescriptions than to fully evaluate how effective existing ones may be and consider removing them. Educate yourself about all the drugs you take and have periodic in-depth reviews of them with your doctor

Your healthcare is just that: yours. Be an active participant and remember that you have the final say. As much as you may love, admire, and respect your healthcare professionals, remember that they are working for you instead of the other way around. You know best how *you* feel and are perfectly capable of learning enough about conditions and drugs from the most legitimate sources on your own that you should demand honest, non-condescending discussions of your own treatment plan.

4 YOU WON'T DIE OF *NOTHING*

You're going to die, and it will probably be sooner than it has been. But there are things you can do to make the time you have left better.

There's nothing better than a ripe pear. I mean very ripe, not still green and hard the way they often come from the grocery. Get one fresh from the tree and it will often have a couple little brownish spots where it's been poked by limbs. It may be slightly bruised on one side, where it fell from the tree or someone squeezed too hard while picking it. Set it on the sill for a couple of days and the skin begins to brown slightly, and those small past traumas become more pronounced. Sometimes it still looks pretty good on the outside, but at the core it's gone to mush. But at just the right moment, at that delectable cosmic intersection of prematurity and decay, it's magical. There's nothing sweeter.

You're that pear. The only thing that will stop the progression of your physical deterioration is for you to die and it completes itself. It's predictable, expected, inevitable, and even welcome in some circumstances. You can do things to slow the negative effects of aging and make the most of life despite them. The first step is understanding what's likely to happen, and how best to deal with it.

Not everyone will experience every problem, and some won't wait until they are seniors to suffer or even die from them. Your lifestyle, genetics, and so many other factors will determine much of it, though sometimes it appears to be just plain luck, good or bad. We will begin by talking about the most serious maladies, one or a combination of which is likely to eventually take you out, according to the U.S. Department of Health and Human Services Centers for Disease Control and Prevention (CDC). All too often these things aren't explained to us in context and how they relate to one another.

Do not get paranoid or depressed. Yes, unless you step in front of a bus, something in this chapter is most likely going to kill you. As we will see, many of them are so interconnected that whatever is written on your death certificate will really be just one part of a multilayered cascade of organ and system failures that are probably inevitable.

Besides, do you really want to be known for having died of *nothing*? Everybody deserves at least that degree of individuality, to have died of *something*, even if that something has been shared by billions over the centuries.

HEART DISEASE:

Some of you reading this probably tell people you have had a heart attack, and many of us know people who died from them. That's a very imprecise term, and there is a wide range of heart ailments that can cause disability and death. There are really three distinct facets of heart function: the pumps (the two sides of the heart), the pipes, and the electrical system. The right pump receives blood from the body and then pushes it to the lungs to pick up oxygen. The left side gets that blood back from the lungs and pumps it on through the whole body, from brain to toes. Along the way, the blood all gets filtered by various organs and forced through vessels big and small, using up that oxygen before making it back into the right pump to begin the process again. The pumps themselves often cannot beat as fast during exertion as they once did after we age, so our performance declines and we get out of breath more easily. Our resting heartrate is less prone to change over the years. Passages in the heart can clog up with fat and calcium, and valves opening and closing the chambers can fray around the edges and deteriorate. The muscle itself can get large and flabby and inefficient.

Pipe problems are plumbing obstructions of the arteries. They become stiff and inflexible over time, called *arteriosclerosis*, or hardening of the arteries. If the arteries are less flexible, the heart must pump harder to force the blood through (high blood pressure in other words) and circulation suffers. *Atherosclerosis* is a specific variety of arteriosclerosis in which the insides of the vessels get constricted by a buildup of that fat and calcium and cellular debris gunk similar to what you would find stuck in the trap of your bathroom sink.

Electrical troubles are a bit harder to understand. You've got four receiving/pumping actions going on all at once, two on the left side and two on the right side. It all must work in unison or blood gets squeezed places it shouldn't go or stays places it shouldn't languish. All this is orchestrated through nerves and tiny electrical stimuli. You could have a perfectly healthy, strong, and robust heart muscle with a screwed up electrical system that doesn't coordinate all the actions which could, at its worst, cause sudden death. Heartbeats that are too fast, slow, or irregular caused by electrical problems are called *arrhythmias*. One of the most common is called *atrial fibrillation*, or "A-Fib." More on these later.

Now, what makes all this so difficult to understand (even for me, and I used to be a biology teacher!) is that these things are so completely integrated. A problem with any of the three components can be caused by the other two and will in turn cause additional trouble for one another. Let's sort out some of the different terms and then talk about how these things most commonly affect us.

Angina – Chest pain that occurs when diseased blood vessels restrict blood flow to the heart. I will not regale you with the old naughty joke about a misunderstood diagnosis of *acute angina* being mistaken for a compliment here, but if we ever meet in person and you buy me a couple of beers, I may be persuaded.

Angioplasty - Briefly inflating a tiny balloon inside an artery to open it up, done with a thin device called a balloon catheter.

Arrhythmia - An abnormal heartbeat. When your heart flutters, quivers, skips beats, or feels like it's banging out of your chest, it may indicate Atrial fibrillation, or A-Fib. Instead of contracting and relaxing to a regular pattern, the heart upper chambers, or atria, beat irregularly, not pushing enough blood out and allowing it to pool.

Blood clot – A glob of thick blood. They are beneficial when they stop the flow of blood from an injury, but they can also form inside an artery when the artery's walls are damaged and cause a heart attack or stroke.

Bradycardia – A slow heartbeat.

Bypass – Surgery that reroutes blood flow around a section of clogged or diseased artery. Often a section of healthy blood vessel from your leg is grafted onto the left main heart artery that supplies blood to the heart muscle itself.

Cardiac arrest – The heart stops, usually because of electrical signal disruption, suddenly and often without warning. (Compare this to Heart Attack below)

Catheterization – Often called a "heart cath," inserting a fine, hollow tube into an artery, usually in the groin, and passing the tube into the heart, allowing the doctor to observe it, take measurements, look for clots and damage, and even take tissue samples. It's usually done while you are awake.

Cardiovascular Disease - Or just "heart disease," a general term that can include coronary artery disease, valve disease, arrhythmia, peripheral vascular disease, congenital heart defects, hypertension, and cardiomyopathy.

Congestive heart failure - When the heart cannot pump all the blood returning to it, the blood backs up in the vessels and there is an accumulation of fluid in the body's tissues, including the lungs. Swollen ankles and legs (edema) can be a sign of CHF.

Coronary heart disease – A buildup of atherosclerotic plaque in the coronary arteries causing blockages that can lead to angina or heart attack.

Electrocardiogram (ECG or EKG) – A test in which electronic sensors are placed on the body to monitor electrical activity associated with the heartbeat. It's painless.

Enlarged heart – When the heart is larger than normal. There are many causes, including heredity or long-term heavy exercise, or disorders like obesity, high blood pressure, and coronary artery disease.

Heart attack – Damage to part of the heart (or the entire thing if severe enough) muscle caused by a lack of oxygen-rich blood flowing to it. The more technical medical term is *myocardial infarction*, or MI. We visualize the stereotype of clutching one's chest and slumping over (which certainly does sometime happen), but there can also be mild cases you hardly notice, sometimes called "silent heart attacks." You may think it's regular heartburn or a strained muscle. It may still be damaging, and whatever caused it may strike again as a killer. Warning signs of heart attack include the classic chest and/or left arm pain but may also manifest in other upper body discomfort (jaw or back), shortness of breath, lightheadedness, nausea, or vomiting. (Compare this to Cardiac Arrest above)

Ischemia – Decreased blood flow to the heart, usually due to a constricted or blocked artery.

Palpitation – An irregular heartbeat that you can feel.

Plaque – A deposit of gunk in the inner lining of the artery wall in atherosclerosis.

Stent – A tiny, expandable, metal mesh that is placed in a narrowing artery by using a catheter and left in place to keep the artery open.

Stress Test – Evaluating the heart while it is being worked. This will often be done while running of a treadmill, or, if you can't do that, given drugs to raise your heart rate. Occasionally looking at the "Patient Portion" of your hospital bill might suffice.

Remember our *Pump, Pipe, Electrical* discussion model. Different treatments target different conditions, but they all still end up affecting one another. We'll start with the pump, the heart muscle itself. Two commonly prescribed classes of drugs designed to help the heart work better are ACE inhibitors and Beta-blockers. They ease swelling and fluid buildup and widen arteries so the heart can get the same amount of pumping done with less strain.

Many of you may already be on a drug to help keep the pipes

from clogging. Statins, or anti-cholesterol medications, are some of the most prescribed in the country, with around 80 million people, or a third of all adults, either already or medically eligible to be taking them. Calcium channel blockers and beta blockers lower blood pressure and can slow the heart rate. Remember that A-Fib allows blood to pool in the upper chambers of the heart because it isn't being pumped out efficiently. The problem with pooled blood is that it clots (think about the dark red blob that forms when you cut your finger).

Stated simply, blood clots kill. They become lodged somewhere, shut off blood supply, and you die. If they travel to the brain, you have a stroke; if to the lungs, it's a pulmonary embolism. That's why A-Fib calls for a blood thinner, to keep pooled or poorly circulating blood from clotting. More than 8 million Americans take blood thinners, and must be aware that, while helping prevent fatal clots, they also cause one to bleed more readily. A cut can become more serious, and bruises, caused by small amounts of blood being spilled just under the skin's surface, more common.

So many things to go wrong, with stakes so high! But your heart begins beating long before you are a recognizable human in the womb and will do so about 2.5 billion times before it quits. Heart disease is so complicated because it both affects and is affected by so many other things, such as diabetes, kidney function, alcohol, smoking, diet, physical activity, heredity, and just about everything else involved in the human condition. Maladies of the heart can take you on a slow, debilitating journey from activity to being bedridden, or can cause you to wake up in the middle of the night after a perfectly normal day and literally drop dead in the bathroom while looking for some Tums.

What about taking a daily low dose aspirin to help prevent heart attacks? The guidance has evolved a bit over the years, and there are some "depending on who you ask" differences. They are often based on your other cardiac risk factors vs. your risk of gastrointestinal hemorrhage. Remember that no drug, not even aspirin, is without side effects. Aspirin does thin the blood, so if you have a ruptured aneurysm, it could mean the difference between having a few minutes to get emergency treatment and, well, not having them. The inevitable "broken record" statement in this chapter is to discuss it with your doctor.

Speaking of broken records: Did I mention eating a balanced, healthy diet, getting plenty of exercise, maintaining a healthy weight, giving up smoking, using alcohol only moderately, and controlling hypertension, diabetes, and cholesterol? It won't be the last you hear of these, as you can probably guess.

HIGH BLOOD PRESSURE:

Hypertension isn't really separate from heart disease and is so common that almost a third of the American adult population has had physicians recommend medication for it. When the force of blood against your artery walls is too high, your heart must work much harder to keep it flowing. And, just like water through a hose, pressure that is too high can cause arteries to bulge (an aneurysm) and rupture, causing death.

Heredity, lifestyle, stress, smoking, and diet all affect it, just like interconnected heart disease, but with many people there is no identifiable underlying cause. It's measured on a millimeters of mercury (mm Hg) scale and includes both the pressure when the heart pumps (systolic, or upper number) and when it is at rest (diastolic, or lower number). While "normal" is a relative term, the target for healthy blood pressure is 120/80 or lower. Your blood pressure is considered elevated it your upper number is 120-129 AND your lower number is still 80 or lower. Stage 1 hypertension is diagnosed with an upper number of 130-139 OR a lower number from 80-89 (note the shift from AND to OR). Stage 2 hypertension is diagnosed with an upper number of 140 or higher OR a lower number of 90 or higher.

You may exhibit some symptoms from high blood pressure, such as headaches, nosebleeds, or shortness of breath, or you may not and have no clue anything is wrong. There are several things that are rightfully called "silent killers," and this is one of them. If hypertension is mild when first diagnosed, a doctor may suggest trying lifestyle changes first, including a better diet with low sodium, exercise, losing weight, reducing alcohol and eliminating smoking, adequate sleep, and reducing stress. (I mean, it's really kind of hard to argue with any of those for any ailment, right?) The first treatment is often a diuretic, or "water pill." They remove sodium and water from your body through increased urination. Sit on the bench outside the men's room at Walmart long enough and one will likely hear older gentlemen badmouthing those "darn water pills." Since this also often reduces the potassium in the blood (necessary to regulate heartbeat), it's important to keep those levels checked when taking diuretics. ACE inhibitors may also be prescribed, and they work differently, blocking the formation of natural chemicals that narrow the blood vessels. There are several anti-hypertension medications called "blockers," "antagonists," "vasodilators," and "inhibitors," and sometimes it takes trial and error to find what combination works best for an individual.

My friends and family know me as a science guy, research driven, an INTJ, and generally boring to others not so inclined. They may be surprised by my inclusion of the next item, but there is good science behind it: Mindfulness, Meditation, and Biofeedback can, for many, be an effective part of hypertension treatment, so much so that even more enlightened health insurance companies are beginning to recognize it. Relaxation and meditation techniques have been widely studied and found to be effective by, among others, the Harvard-affiliated Benson-Henry Institute for Mind Body Medicine.

It makes sense, when you think about it: stress causes adrenaline to flow, increasing blood pressure and heart rate. In our ancient past, that was necessary to run away from saber toothed tigers, but today we sit and grumble instead of using up that adrenaline to run. That extra blood pressure turns inward. These techniques can lower stress, thus lowering blood pressure. It's not as easy as taking a pill but could have untold additional benefits.

DIABETES (with a side of CHOLESTOROL):

Okay, I probably do pronounce it like the late actor Wilford Brimley did. But, hey, he's the dead celebrity who I most resemble physically, so why not?

You already know the condition is caused by blood sugar levels being too high. Pharmaceutical commercials and people who want to sound fancy often used the term "A1C," which is simply the name for a test that measures your blood sugar levels over time, often three months. The normal range is below 5.7%, from there up to 6.4% is considered "prediabetic," and 6.5% or higher gives you a diabetic diagnosis.

The "less bad" news is that only around 0.55% of Americans have Type I "born this way" diabetes. (No disrespect, of course, for that's still substantial number of people. They often must take insulin injections their entire life and may suffer heart and kidney damage.) The true epidemic is in the explosion of Type II ("adult onset") diabetes. About 1 in 10 Americans are diabetic with 90-95% of those being Type II (Centers for Disease Control statistics), but for those 65 and older, that number raises to almost 1 in 3. As we get plumper and less active as a society and there are more overweight children and teens, the onset of Type II diabetes occurs at younger and younger ages.

High blood sugar is not caused by a problem with the blood itself. It's a one-two punch involving the pancreas and what happens metabolically within the cells and systems. The pancreas does not produce enough insulin to process sugar, and the body becomes resistant to the insulin that is being produced. This causes cells in the muscles and fatty tissue and liver to not take in sugar efficiently, so it gets recirculated in the blood instead. (Many of us educated in the 1960s and 1970s remember laboring to spell "Islets of Langerhans" in biology class. These are the tiny clusters of cells in the pancreas that do the hormone-producing work, and there are about a million of them per pancreas.) When too much glucose circulates in your blood, it causes long-term harm to tissues, organs, and systems. Your body tries to compensate by making you thirsty so you will urinate more. Nerve damage can cause tingling and numbness in your extremities, and sores are slow to heal. Over time, you may develop gangrenous ulcers and loss of circulation that may even require limb amputation, plus vision loss, and heart and kidney damage.

It's not a good road, but the chances of older folks walking it for at least part of their lives are high and getting higher. The prestigious Mayo Clinic lists the following factors that may increase the risk of Type II diabetes:

-*Being obese or overweight.* For some reason, where one carries that extra weight makes a difference. If in the abdomen (commonly the case for men) instead of the hips or thighs, the risk is greater. Specifically, if a man has a waist circumference more than 40 inches or a women more than 35 inches, be warned. And, brothers, 40 inches does not mean where you wear your pants because you have worn a 38-inch groove in your abdomen over the past half century. Pull 'em up (if you can) until your black nylon dress socks are fully visible in those Crocs and you will see what I mean.

-*Inactivity.* Exercise uses up that extra glucose as fuel. Burn enough of it and there is less left to cause problems. An active person is also less likely to be obese.

-*Being non-Caucasian.* It's unclear why, but statistically significant.

-*Being 35+* (raises hand).

-*Having a family history of the disease.*

There are other blood chemistry factors as well, and this is where diabetes and the dreaded "high cholesterol" intersect. Like many bodily functions, they are so interconnected that maladies must often be medically treated as a system rather than individual conditions. You have probably heard of "good" and "bad" cholesterol, HDL and LDL, but who other than a healthcare professional or annoying know-it-all can remember which is which? Then there are *triglycerides* which are like the 70s stoners wanting to get high and are different but still connected, or something?

In a nutshell: cholesterol and triglycerides are both *lipids*, or fatty acids, that circulate in our blood. They are natural and necessary for metabolism but can get out of whack. There are two main types of cholesterol: High-density lipoprotein (HDL) and Low-density lipoprotein, or LDL. A blood test may give you a total cholesterol number (HDL+LDL+triglycerides) preferably under 200 mg/dl), but it's important to know the breakdown in a lipid panel. The HDL is often called "good cholesterol" because it picks up other cholesterol from the blood and carries it back to the liver for processing. It's preferable to have an HDL reading of 55 mg/dl or more for women and 45 mg/dl or more for men.

The LDL, or "bad cholesterol," on the other hand, delivers itself to the cells but is too lazy to carry any excess back to the liver, instead just depositing it on the blood vessel walls. This causes atherosclerosis, like that old, galvanized pipe under the sink that barely lets any water through anymore, and a blob of corrosion can break off and travel around until it clogs up something very important. Bad. It's best for your LDL to be under 100 mg/dl.

Then the triglycerides come in to further complicate things. These blood fats are less "waxy" than cholesterols and are both produced by the body itself and consumed, especially in meat and plant oils. A healthy triglyceride number is 150 mg/dl or less; higher numbers put you at risk for not only heart and blood vessel disease, but Type II diabetes.

Did I mention it's all so interconnected?

Now the good news: while much of this is genetic, most people can positively affect their risk of Type II diabetes with lifestyle changes, including a healthy diet, weight loss, and exercise.

And the bad news: that requires *actually* eating a healthy diet, losing weight, and exercising. But the effect can be dramatic. In fact, while reluctant to use the word "cure," putting the disease "in remission" for the rest of your life may, indeed, be possible. Several studies, including those funded by Diabetes UK, have confirmed just that.

While lifestyle change is difficult and takes time to show effect, popping a pill is easier and more immediate. But every medication can have drawbacks. They may not work for everyone, can be expensive, and become less effective over time. Nonetheless, we live in a world of upbeat pharmaceutical commercials and seem to look to pills and injections as the first resort rather than the last. The initial prescription is often metformin, which reduces the amount of glucose produced by the liver. Some folks can take it with hardly noticing any side effects at all, while others have such gastrointestinal distress that they discontinue it. After that front-line prescription, there is a whole range of other inhibitors and antagonists designed to reduce blood glucose levels.

But is the game about to change? If losing weight can put the disease into remission, what about treating it with a drug to just *lose weight*? In addition to Type II diabetes, that could have a host of other positive health effects, not to mention looking better nekked, as we Appalachians say.

Has the age-old dream finally been realized? Semaglutide, dulaglutide, liraglutide, tirzepatide and similar drugs have been big news ever since first approved as Type II diabetes treatments and some now directly for weight loss even without being diabetic. They are known as *incretin mimetics* and were first inspired by Gila monster venom. I'm not kidding. They work not by specifically lowering blood sugar or fat or anything else, but rather slowing the progression of food from the stomach into the small intestine. You feel full faster, and for longer, so you eat less. It still all boils down to that, and thus your risk factors for diabetes, hypertension, kidney failure, heart disease, and many other things dissipate.

Of course, there are side effects that vary widely from person to person, as does the amount of weight loss. They are expensive, and not always covered by health insurance either fully or even partially. And to maintain the weight loss, you may have to take the medications indefinitely.

But still…are we on the verge of being able to conquer the first world epidemic of obesity with all its attendant diseases? Or will only rich people be able to do so? Half the world suffers from too much food and too little exercise, while the other half suffers from just the opposite. Can't we just summons the will power to do what we know we need to do to stay healthy? Sadly, no. Only about 20% of Americans who lose weight can keep it off long term (Wing, Rena and Phelan, Suzanne. Long-term weight loss maintenance, *National Library of Medicine*, July 2005. I believe I met Dr. Wing once during my 20-year stint as a diabetes prevention study participant at the University of Pittsburgh. Since I was often at the sharp end of a needle, I never wore any of my West Virginia University ball cap or jacket for those visits).

The ultimate option for otherwise uncontrolled diabetes, of course, is daily insulin injections. While they may eventually become as routine for those taking them as brushing teeth, they control your schedule and require you to think about things like refrigerator access and meal timing. But compared to hugging your oxygen tank while being pushed in a wheelchair because you no longer have legs and going three times a week to dialysis and hoping the person driving you is going to the right place because you are blind, it seems like a bargain. I know that is stark; bleak, even. But uncontrolled diabetes can do all those things to you. Even with intervention, the effects eventually take their toll. Far too many times I have heard older people say things like, "Oh, the doctor gave me a pill for sugar, but I'm going to eat what I want. If it ain't killed me yet, it ain't goin' to now." With work, there are things you can do to help stave off, or at least delay, the full-body debilitation brought on by diabetes. Do what you want, but someone will have to be paid to push that wheelchair if you delay.

I didn't say I am here to make you feel good about things, now did I?

CANCER:

There. I said it. We've all seen it, we all fear it, and around half of us will have some sort of it in our lifetime (Cancer Research UK {www.cruk.org}). That is a chilling statement, but in mitigation remember that we are living longer and cancer risks increase with age. Many cancers are not only treatable but completely curable, and some are so slow that we just live with them until we don't anymore. And, while it can't be precisely figured, it's estimated that up to 40% of cancers are preventable with healthy lifestyle changes. There's THAT again! There are more than 100 types of cancer that affect humans, so generalization isn't always helpful, but cancer occurs when cells, for some reason, begin reproducing abnormally. Like the monster from the old sci-fi film *The Blob*, they grow and begin to invade the other cells, forming tumors and spreading through whatever path presents itself. This new cancerous tissue doesn't perform its intended function and supplants healthy tissue. Tumors can become unbelievably huge without treatment, practically filling up whole body cavities. Cancerous cells can travel through the blood or lymphatic systems to infect new areas. Growth can be swift, or it can be "watchful waiting" decades long.

About 2 million Americans are newly diagnosed with some form of cancer each year. According to the American Cancer Society (Atlanta, Georgia 2023), breast cancer is by far the most common type for women, and prostate for men. The next two most common for both sexes are lung and colon. Uterine cancer comes in fourth place for women and bladder cancer for men. Skin cancer is next for both sexes. Almost half of all actual deaths from cancer come from (in order) lung, colon, pancreas, and breast cancers.

Most types of cancer are so much more treatable and survivable and beatable today than just a few years ago. In fact, a new diagnosis is about twice as survivable as it was when you and I were teens. There are many new types of drugs almost unfathomable to our grandparents' generation when there was little to do but remove tumors if they could be reached and hope for the best. The dialog from the John Wayne/Jimmy Stewart western *The Shootist* wasn't far from the mark. Stewart, as Doctor E. W. Hostetler, gives the Duke's character John Bernard Books the bad news: he has cancer. "Can't you cut it out, Doc?" asks Books. "I'd have to gut you like a fish," replies Hostetler. (*The Shootist*, Paramount Pictures, 1976. Screenplay by Miles Hood Swarthout. It was, ironically, Wayne's final film before his death in 1979...of cancer. The film had an incredible cast. Wayne's last appearance, at the 1979 Academy Awards ceremony, is available on YouTube, and is very difficult to watch, at least for me).

There can be a genetic predisposition for various cancers. It's important that your doctor know your family history with the disease a couple of generations back. Lifestyle and environmental factors like chemicals and ultraviolet radiation are also huge. But simply being around for a long while increases your risk, almost as if it is a natural state for old folks. Cell damage builds up, and sometimes the new ones just start acting differently, no longer playing by the old rules. Let's look at some specifics about the most common types of cancer.

Breast

The breast is made up of milk-producing glands called *lobules*, ducts that carry milk to the nipple, and lots of fatty and fibrous connective tissue holding everything together. Most cancers begin in either the lobules or ducts, though there are a few rarer types. From either place, the cancer can spread, or *metastasize*, into the rest of the breast and then throughout the body. Sometimes there are no symptoms or signs at all before the cancer spreads, and different people may have very different symptoms. But, straight from the CDC, here are warning signs to look for:

- A lump in the breast or armpit
- Thickening or swelling in any part of the breast
- Irritation or dimpling of the breast skin
- Redness or flaky skin in the nipple area
- Pulling in of the nipple or pain in the nipple area
- Nipple discharge, including blood
- Any change in the size or shape of the breast, or
- Pain in any area of the breast

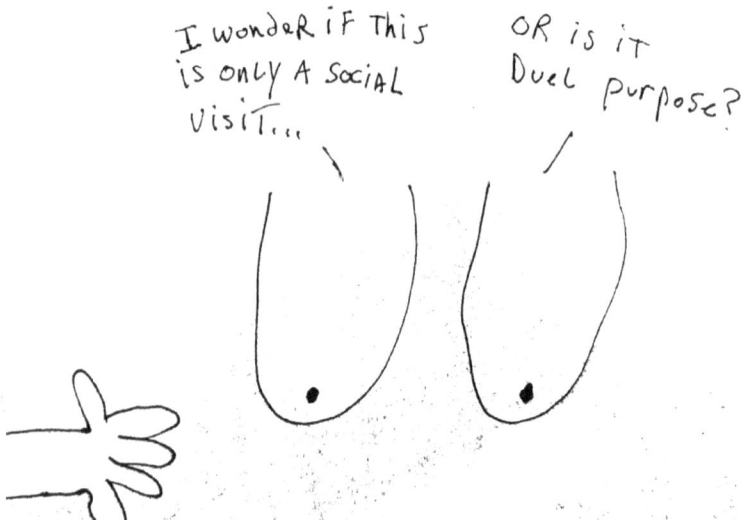

Examine yourself often. I am not being naughtily suggestive in any way here, but train your partner, if you have one, to help you. Sometimes someone else notices things we do not. It is beyond irony that a young man so eager to touch the breasts of the object of his affection may be uncomfortable doing so with purpose in later years when it can be of such importance. Grow up whydontcha.

Finding a lump does not necessarily mean cancer. Many are benign. Unfortunately, both women and men may notice something and avoid seeking medical attention out of fear, allowing time for the cancer, if indeed present, to spread. That is a very human response, but denial is the worst possible strategy. In addition to regular self-exams, the United States Preventive Services Task Force recommends women 50-74 at average risk (no prior or close family history of breast cancer or other enhanced risk factors) get a mammogram every two years. Beginning at age 40, women should discuss risks vs. potential benefits with their doctors.

What happens if something is questionable? In addition to a mammogram, other diagnostic tools are available, such as an ultrasound, MRI, and, ultimately, a biopsy, in which fluid or tissue is removed and examined for cancer cells. If they are found, further tests will be conducted to see the extent of spread. This is called *staging*, determining to what stage the cancer has progressed. It's more complicated than a simple "Stage 1-3" or similar designation.

The type and stage of cancer will determine treatment options. It may require a mastectomy, or breast removal. Depending on the size of the tumor and spread, much of the breast tissue may be saved, but sometimes it cannot, and the entire breast, duct system, and even underlying tissue must be removed. Reconstructive procedures may be part of the surgery. Other therapies can also be used. Radiation will either be administered by a machine outside the body in treatment sessions or through pellets implanted directly into or near the cancer. Chemotherapy and hormone therapy drugs are either injected or given orally.

I don't have to tell you, of course, that there are often unpleasant side effects to these therapies, but treatments to help mitigate some of them exist. A newer treatment called targeted therapy uses monoclonal antibodies designed to trigger the body's own immune system to attack the cancer. There has been great progress, and research continues, promising more weapons against this disease soon.

A mastectomy is major surgery, and a thorough recovery period of carefully following instructions, including how long to wait before wearing a breast prosthesis or bra, is necessary.

Hormone exposure can affect one's breast cancer risk. If you had early periods and late menopause you were exposed to estrogen and other hormones longer. Hormone replacement therapy can do the same thing. As to things you can change, all the lifestyle choices for reducing cancer risk in general apply to breast cancer as well.

Finally, almost everything in this section can also apply to men. It's little discussed, but almost 3,000 American men are diagnosed with breast cancer per year, and more than 500 will die from it. One wonders how many of those deaths would have been preventable with early detection and treatment. While men may be aware (and promptly ignore) that they should do regular testicular self-exams, the same caution for male breast exams is widely unknown.

Prostate

We never seem to think about the wee guy until he starts causing us problems, kind of like our doorbell transformer or car's voltage regulator. I have read many descriptions of the prostate over the years, and almost all of them compare its size and shape to a walnut. It sits just under the bladder and the urethra runs through it. This little gland produces a fluid that nourishes the sperm for their arduous journey up the cervix and uterus to the oviduct (or a handy 1970s tube sock with blue and gold stripes on top ready for the next day's laundry, whichever the case may have been for 1970s you. Fashions change), essentially packing a lunch for those microscopic warriors intent on continuing the species. There is a misconception (no pun) that pre-ejaculate (who calls it that *ever*?) released before the main event originates in the prostate, but that is not the case. That clear-ish fluid is produced by accessory sex glands, with glorious names like Cowper's Gland, the Glands of Littre, and the Glands of Morgagni. (Why do those names remind me of the *Lord of the Rings?*)

Brethren, your chances of getting prostate cancer are excellent if you are fortunate enough to live a long life. About 13 out of a hundred guys will be diagnosed with it, and a couple will die from it. But that is not an age-weighted statistic and counts only formal diagnosis. This number is more telling: about 80% of men who reach the age of 80 have cancer cells in their prostate. 80 and 80. Wow. Black men are more at risk, and a family history of prostate, pancreatic, or ovarian cancer raise the chances as well, plus all the environmental factors associated with other types of cancer.

And get this: compared to men who ejaculate 4 to 7 times per month across their lifetimes, men who ejaculated 21 or more times a month have a 31% LOWER risk of prostate cancer! WHO SAYS I ONLY HAVE BAD NEWS? Stay mission driven, and results focused, guys! (And no, I didn't make that up. It comes from the Harvard Ejaculation Study, part of the officially dubbed *Health Professionals Follow-Up Study*, which followed almost 30,000 men from 1992 through 2000. You mean you haven't read it?).

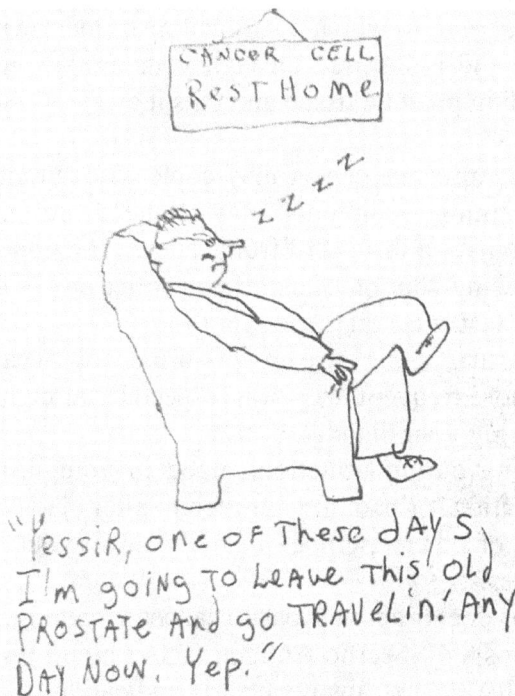

"Yessir, one of these days, I'm going to leave this old prostate and go travelin' any day now. Yep."

Prostate cancers are not all created equal, though. The younger you are when diagnosed, the more likely it is for you to have a more aggressive, fast-growing type. Generally, the older you are, the less aggressive it often is, especially if you are 70+. It's like the cancer cells are sitting around in the prostate common room talking about going on a trip someday but not really finding the energy to do so. "Yeah, I would like to go check out the lymph nodes, but I don't drive at night anymore." Even if it is aggressive, prostate cancer is one of the most curable, provided it's treated early.

Even if you never have cancer, other prostate issues are likely to come your way. Unlike some pension checks, the prostate very often gets bigger with age, and that walnut becomes a lemon, partially blocking off your urine stream. You may have to stand quite a while to get the flow started, and even then, it's weak, and you may not feel your bladder completely empties. It can get so bad that it practically cuts off urination completely, which can be fatal. There are drugs to counteract this, but sometimes removal of even non-cancerous prostates can become necessary. More common, though, is a *transurethral resection*, in which a surgical instrument with an electrical loop at the end is inserted through your urethra until it encounters the offending prostate tissue and cuts it away. Keep that happy thought.

Like many cancers, prostate cancer may come with symptoms, or without, and common symptoms may come from simple enlargement or inflammation instead of from cancer. The important thing is to not delay seeing your physician if you notice any of them, even between regular visits. Be on the lookout for:

Difficulty starting your stream of urine, or weak or interrupted flow or more frequent urination (especially at night), or not completely emptying your bladder.

Pain or burning during urination, blood in your urine or semen, painful ejaculation (or pain in your rectum after ejaculation, a sign of prostatitis), or otherwise unexplained pain in your back, hips, or pelvis that persists.

Talk with your doctor about prostate cancer screening. That usually involves a Prostate Specific Antigen (PSA) blood test. Be aware that PSA results are not always clearly indicative, though, because various things can affect the levels, and that's why there aren't necessarily "set" levels as a norm, though something around 4.0 ng/ml or lower is sometimes used. A higher number may indicate additional tests are needed, or simply testing again soon, along with a digital exam. No, that doesn't mean the exam is more advanced than analog: a healthcare professional lubes up his or her latex-gloved finger and inserts in into your rectum to feel your prostate for anything abnormal. (Oh, stop being such a wimp. Compared to a typical gynecological exam, that's nothing.)

If there is still a more aggressive diagnostic procedure needed, you may have a biopsy. In the most common type, you will self-administer an enema the night before, go to the surgical center, and have an IV inserted. You will be given a sedative and a local anesthetic, but whether you are fully asleep depends on several health factors as well as your physician's decisions. You will lay on your side with bent knees while he or she inserts a device through your rectum into your prostate, guided by ultrasound. The device is spring-loaded and with a *click-click-click* extracts several tissue samples from various areas of your prostate, to be examined in the lab for cancer cells. Easy peasy. You will feel sore for a while, of course, and there may be small amounts of blood in your urine and stool for several days. A more disturbing sight for men not expecting it is blood in the semen, turning it a gosh-awful nasty rust color. And that could persist to some degree for a month or more!

Guys being guys, we expect that, if any cancer cells are found, it's time to cry "Havoc!" and let slip the dogs of war against the prostate, ending your long (and previously productive) association completely by ripping it out. Not so fast! Unless the cancer is of an aggressive nature, the more likely recommendation will be one of "watchful waiting." In other words, you and your physician patiently monitor the cancer that isn't causing any symptoms over the long term, avoiding treatment unless it begins to spread or cause other problems. I know "patiently" may not be a term often applied to us guys, especially when anything groin-related in involved, but the fact is that many prostate cancers grow so slowly and cause so few symptoms that it is riskier to do something than to do nothing. The rest of your body may happily get old and die while those cancer cells are still in that common room watching Rick Steves but never leaving their recliners. In fact, some guidelines now discourage men at only average risk from even being routinely screened past the age 70 unless there are symptoms. (Here's where I am allowed to say I plan to make a different personal choice and will continue to get screened annually. Talk with your doctor.)

Untreated, aggressive prostate cancer spreads into the surrounding tissues and organs and can kill. The options are somewhat like those with breast cancer, including surgery, radiation, chemo, and immunotherapy. Like any invasive procedure, treatment will have side effects. After prostate removal, roughly 1 in 5 men may be left with some degree of urinary or erectile dysfunction. Resuming sexual activity as soon as possible after the procedure may help prevent irreversible erectile dysfunction (Schout, Barbara and Meuleman, Eric. Erectile dysfunction and incontinence after prostatectomy, *Urologie,* Amsterdam, the Netherlands, 2012), so man up and take one for the team ASAP.

Colon

Just like Type II diabetes, colon (or colorectal) cancer is increasingly being seen in relatively young and otherwise healthy people, like the exceptionally talented actor Chadwick Boseman, who battled the disease for four years and died at only 43. Tragic. Like with other cancers, early detection is the key. Colon cancer begins when cells go haywire in the lining, forming little clumps called *polyps.* Some polyps aren't cancerous at all, but they are where the trouble usually begins, and it can take a decade or longer for a polyp to become cancerous. Sometimes a particularly insidious one can spread more quickly. One obvious warning sign is blood in your stool, but there are other things, such as hemorrhoids, that can cause that as well. Other signs can include changes in bowel habits, abdominal pain, unexplained weight loss, or anemia, all of which can have causes other than cancer.

The only way to make sure is to be tested. The most common diagnostic tool, a colonoscopy, has the added advantage of being preventive as well, because polyps can be removed during the procedure. Increasingly popular in lower risk individuals with no family history is the much-advertised DNA test, that searches small samples of your stool for signs of cancerous cell mutations.

My wife was the first of us to do the mail-in colon cancer test. The white box used to return the sample is nondescript, I guess, but obvious if you are familiar with it. So she did the logical thing: she sent me to the UPS store to ship it. I went early, so I could be at the store when it opened and not stand in line. In fact, there was only one other person ahead of me at the counter, a guy about my age…holding an identical white box!

Hey, if heartthrob Harry Connick Jr. can do it with pride, so can you. Harry's wife is a breast cancer survivor; they are tireless advocates of early cancer screening and I salute them for it. It's easy, completely painless, and less unpleasant than changing an older baby's diaper.

It's not for everyone, though. If your risk factors are higher, your doctor will likely suggest the colonoscopy route. Get over your dread. A study by researchers at the Cleveland Clinic (29) found two-thirds of patients reported "little or no" pain. I suspect a newer study would find an even higher "little or no" stat, with more advanced techniques. You will receive anesthesia, and sedation is seldom even necessary. I have known someone who died of colon cancer, a World War II vet who I greatly respected, and it's not a good way to go. Any testing discomfort, real or only feared, is worth the peace of mind.

Surgery is still the most common treatment for colon cancer, but others, such as chemo and radiation, are also in the toolkit. If that sounds like a repeat of other cancer treatments in the sections above, it is. So is the list of things you can do to help prevent it. The "eat a healthy diet" item on that list includes lots of fiber, preferably in the form of fresh vegetables and fruits and whole grains.

The recommendation for beginning testing for colon cancer through whichever means recommended by one's doctor was once age 50. It is now 45. Do it.

Skin

Yep, I'm in on this one. A little spot on my left forehead (which is, shall we say, much more exposed these days than it was in years past) started growing both suddenly and quickly. My RN wife noticed it while we were on vacation and stated flatly that I was to see a dermatologist ASAP. A biopsy revealed squamous cell carcinoma, a common type of skin cancer mostly caused by ultraviolet radiation. I grew up working on our little farm without ever thinking twice about protection from the sun and have always enjoyed doing things outdoors, so it was really no surprise. The most common types of skin cancer are *Basal cell* that begins deep in the skin in the area where new cells are generated; *Squamous cell* that begins in the middle and outer layers of skin, and *melanoma* that develops in the cells that produce your skin pigment and is the most serious type of skin cancer.

There are many changes in the skin as we age that are completely natural and expected and not cancerous. We get those annoying skin tags, especially where one thing rubs against another, such as underarms, and they can be especially irritating on eyelids...or, in my case, embarrassing during examination by the young female PA where some *parts* rubbed against other of my *parts*. But, if intentionally or accidently plucked off, they can bleed profusely, so it's best to let a professional take care of them with a simple shot of anesthetic, a snip, and a bandage. There are also those permanent bright red spots that pop up, called *cherry angiomas*, which are usually harmless. Aging brings on all manner of warts and sties and pustules and ingrown hairs and "liver spots" and other imperfections showing we have survived not only the disco age but several ages since. Wear them proudly. Baby bottoms are beautifully smooth, but do not announce to the world the wealth of experience we possess.

If there is something new, something growing, something that just doesn't look good, especially on the areas most exposed to the sun, get it checked out. This includes waxy bumps, bleedy scabs, lesions, crusty surfaces, moles that change in any way (including just color), and nodules. Even if it's not time for your regular checkup, see your doctor, or self-refer to a dermatologist. She or he may conduct a full body check and, if there are suspicious areas, schedule a biopsy. While it's often considered cosmetic surgery and therefore not covered by insurance, you may have those pesky skin tags removed at the same time, and inexpensively.

I see my dermatologist annually and visit in between those annual checkups if something seems suspicious and will continue to do so. If you have a family history of skin cancer or you have had any type yourself in the past, it's vitally important that it be continually monitored. Maybe you won't end up like my good friend "J," who sees the same dermatologist as me every six months. It seems like each time the doctor carves on his pale Irish assets. The guy reminds me of the passage in *The Merchant of Venice*, where Shylock tells Bassanio he must "be nominated for an equal pound of your fair flesh, to be cut off and taken." "J" (who, by the way, WAS AT WOODSTOCK when he was 19. How cool is that?) is doing what's necessary to stay ahead of something that could be life threatening if ignored.

Remember that skin cancer can occur where the sun doesn't shine, as well, so don't limit your self-examination to exposed areas. Most of us have, I'll wager, not lived the life of skin cancer prevention. On the contrary, the annual spring sunburn was an adolescent ritual, and even though decades ago increase our chances of cancer today. While we may still love a "healthy tan" gained while sipping our margaritas poolside, we are better off without it. Yes, we do need a healthy dose of Vitamin D synthesized with sun exposure, but the smart move is to cover up and use sun block. UV radiation not only raises cancer risk, but just plain ages your skin, and who needs more of that? I probably shouldn't even mention tanning beds because I don't want my picture hanging in tanning bed manufacturing offices with a target on my forehead, right where that squamous cell cancer scar is still visible.

Pancreatic, lung, esophageal, stomach, bladder, cervical, uterine, and other cancers:

While less common, these are complex and can all be very serious. Early detection is still the key. A more in-depth look at each would far exceed our word count limit, but there are lots of resources available for those wishing (or needing) to understand these types of cancer more fully. Sadly, they sometimes present few recognizable symptoms until the cancer has started spreading. The best catch-all advice is to be aware of changes in your body and not just write them all off as part of getting old, and discussing them with your doctor during regular checkups. This is particularly important if there is any history of cancer in your family, and if (I know this will apply to only a few of you, but I will include it anyway) you haven't led a scrupulously pristine life devoid of eating, drinking, smoking, breathing, or doing the wrong things.

It's not too late to start. Really it isn't. I have heard the "if it ain't hurt me yet" and "it won't do any good now" arguments all my life. They are lies we tell ourselves because we don't want to change. I have served as a pallbearer for more than one friend I have heard use those excuses. As we have seen, one of the only characteristics all these various cancers have in common is a list of things you can do to help prevent them. There is no guarantee because genetics and other factors play such a role but *change what you can change.*

Seven lifestyle choices that can reduce your cancer risk:

-Don't smoke. Duh. Tobacco use accounts for almost a quarter of cancer deaths.

-Keep a healthy weight. Duh.

-Drink only moderate amounts of alcohol. (Enough with the *duhs* already. You get the idea)

-Eat a healthy, high fiber diet and avoid processed meats.

-Lead an active life with plenty of exercise.

-Protect yourself from the sun.

-Protect yourself from carcinogenic chemicals.

I am thinking about leading a seminar on how to incorporate all these things into our lives. It will be held mid-afternoon on the beach in the nude while sitting around a makeshift fire pit roasting weenies, drinking beer, and smoking cigars. $50 a head. Who's with me?

While not cancer prevention, let's add this important early detection strategy (not as well suited for our seminar on the beach) that could well save your life:

-Conduct regular self-examinations, have regular medical checkups with screenings, and report any observed changes, discharges, or abnormalities.

On to another killer:

Stroke

There was a time when, to publicize the warning signs of a

stroke, some in the medical public community started calling it a "brain attack" to capitalize on the familiarity with the term heart attack. It's not that far off, especially in comparison with the *pipes* part of our heart discussion model. Oxygen-carrying blood doesn't get to the brain tissue, and the organ begins to die off as a result. This can be because one of the arteries is blocked by fatty gunk (an *ischemic* stroke), or because it bursts (a *hemorrhagic* stroke). High cholesterol is often the culprit for one, and high blood pressure the other. Ischemic strokes are the most common. I am sure you have heard the term "mini stroke," or TIA (*transient ischemic attack*) as well. This is when the blood flow blockage resolves itself, usually in five minutes or less.

Time lost is brain lost. It's that simple. If you experience stroke symptoms, get to an ER immediately. The two types are treated differently. With an ischemic stroke, you may be given blood thinners and even more powerful "clot busters" to unblock the artery. With a hemorrhagic stroke, it's not hard to see why that same treatment could be disastrous. Instead, drugs to lower the blood pressure until the bleed can be stopped may be used.

Stroke symptoms can mirror those of other things, but they often come on suddenly. They may include trouble walking and balancing, being dizzy, blurred vision, localized numbness or weakness, or trouble speaking or talking. A classic sign is droopiness on one side of the face and slurring, often noticed by others before the person having the stroke. Strange. The NIH and others suggest a way to remember the most common symptoms, called a FAST test:

F-FACE: Ask the person to smile. Does one side of the face droop?

A-ARMS: Ask the person to raise them both. Does one drift downward?

S-SPEECH: Ask the person to repeat a phrase. Is it slurred or confused?

And T-TIME: If any of these symptoms are present, call 911 immediately. The person may (and I am looking in the mirror here) say he or she wants to "just wait to see if it goes away" or ask to be driven instead of calling an ambulance. Don't give in. Treatment can begin as soon as the EMTs arrive, and every second is vital because you are literally losing brain. Be ready for a slew and a half of tests, and treatments can be as simple as injections or as complex as emergency surgery.

About a fourth of people who have a stroke eventually have another one. You may be prescribed drugs to control cholesterol, blood pressure, or diabetes as well as others. Remember that list of lifestyle changes to promote heart health and, for that matter, prevent cancer? Read it again. It gets a lot of mileage. Depending on how much damage was done, physical therapy may be required to recover lost coordination. The brain has remarkable capacity to heal itself, rerouting pathways and learning new ways to do things.

OTHER THINGS TO EXPECT

Little things can become, or lead to, big things. There are natural effects of aging that are inevitable for many of us but still may warrant more than grumbling acceptance because there are therapies to improve them, and diagnostic tools to make sure they aren't indicative of something demanding rapid intervention. This discussion of things that can be exhausting is by no means *exhaustive*.

Balance

That doddering old fool! *Doddering* is a word I read many times and assumed I knew what it meant from context without looking it up, and it worked: moving in a feeble or unsteady way, especially due to being old.

Joints, muscles, and poor eyesight can all lead to doddering, but a major cause as we age is poor balance. It's a vicious circle: poor balance makes us reluctant to move, leading to more poor balance from stiff joints and weak muscles. Many medications can affect balance, as well as inner ear issues, diabetes, heart disease, high blood pressure, and stroke. Adding to the problem is the sad fact that, for many of us, our center of gravity has shifted as we have put on weight, further throwing off our natural gait.

If you begin feeling unsteady, finding the cause is important, so talk with your doctor. If it's one of those causes listed above, there may be something she can do, and it might even uncover other serious concerns that need treatment. On the other hand, if it's mainly because of stiffness and reduced range of motion, more exercise (and losing weight if needed) can often give considerable relief.

One of my favorite "do this right now" suggestions is to, several times a day, simply tiptoe, very slowly, up and down a dozen times or so. Lean forward slightly if it helps with balance while doing it. Feel the burn in you calves. Don't bob…go slowly, especially when coming back down. This strengthens the leg muscles, pumps lazy blood back up to your heart, and is the cheapest, easiest way I know to help improve balance.

If you need a cane or walker to feel comfortable walking, drop your vanity and get one. Invest in a pair of old people shoes with nonskid soles and low heels. Hold on to railings, use the crossings instead of stepping up onto sidewalks, and realize your long relationship with ladders is coming to an end. The more you walk, the more balanced and confident you may become. Walking has so many other benefits that it has its own chapter!

Menopause

Any male who makes jokes about this very real and consequential health condition should fear well deserved cosmic punishment requiring a daily digital prostate exam. Strictly defining menopause's scope is difficult, because it is something that occurs over years with waxing and waning effects. In simple medical terms, it means no longer having periods, and is said to have arrived one year after your last one. All those associated symptoms before that time are known as the menopausal transition, or *perimenopause*. There can be considerable variance, but most women begin it between 45 and 55, and it can go on for more than a decade. Yippee.

The whole thing is triggered by the ovaries ceasing to produce as much of the "female hormones" estrogen and progesterone. They have much more than sexual and reproductive functions, affecting metabolism, bone density and heart health, fat storage, sleep cycles, mental health, temperature regulation, and a host of other things. Some women are fortunate and their bodies adjust to the changes with relative ease, while for a few it can be a true physical and mental health crisis necessitating medical intervention.

If all these things are caused by a lack of female hormones, then just replace them, right? Easy, except it isn't, necessarily. While that works for many women, especially for the symptoms of hot flashes and vaginal dryness, in some cases hormone replacement can increase the risk of blood clots in the legs and lungs, and of breast cancer. You need to weigh out the risks and benefits with a doctor familiar with your personal and family history. There is evidence that counseling or other psychological interventions may have positive outcomes for not just what we consider the emotional and mental concentration consequences of menopause, but even some of the physical, such as hot flashes, as well. (30) There's really no way of knowing what kind of hand menopause will deal you, but don't suffer in silence. It's serious stuff and there are things that can help.

Urinary Issues

An alien observer may think older American earthlings think about urine way too much. An avid tap water and coffee (and should I even mention beer?) drinker, it occupies more of my time than I would like, and I am guilty of the harmful practice of becoming dehydrated while traveling, hoping to reduce bathroom stops. Folks taking diuretics for hypertension also know the score. I have even heard people say, "I want to live as long as I can go to the bathroom by myself, but then I will be ready to die." Is that how little we value our lives?

All muscles atrophy without proper exercise. They can also become stretched or damaged. Incontinence is twice as common in women as men; pregnancy, childbirth, and menopause can be to blame. If the sphincter muscles are weak or the bladder muscles suddenly contract, you may leak urine. If your overall pelvic muscles are not lifting barbells on the beach, they give less support to the whole system. There are medications that may help. Aren't there always? But also consider doing all you can do to strengthen those muscles yourself. The effort may well save some room in your medicine cabinet plus the bonus of maybe, just maybe, feeling good at the same time. Remember the Kegel!

The same exercise that can help tone muscles for more pleasurable sex that we talked about in Chapter 1 strengthens the pelvic floor muscles, thus lending more support to the plumbing. They may help prevent fecal incontinence as well, and improve the symptoms of prolapse, in which the vaginal walls collapse and the organs drop.

You don't have to be left out, guys. Kegels may benefit your incontinence symptoms as well. That comes on the good authority of my own personal urologist, Dr. Irving Patrick Freely. Yep, I. P. and I go back a long way, to junior high school, in fact, along with old friends Willie Makeit and Betty Wont.

Jump on the Kegel bandwagon. None of us are too old to learn new skills, resurrect old ones, and even learn to use new tools, and no new workout clothing or gym memberships are required.

Pneumonia, COPD, and apnea

Reading old death records for genealogy or other research, the "Cause of Death" section tells us a lot about how society has progressed. "Consumption," the archaic word for tuberculosis, took out thousands, as did simple infections that today are easily cured by antibiotics, and the occasional "thrown from horse" and "kicked by mule" add interest. The number of deaths from occupational accidents (I come from a coal mining area) was astounding. And then there was 1918 and the influenza epidemic. Just looking over those old pages is humbling.

One of the Death Parade leaders was pneumonia. Sir William Osler (1849 – 1919), the Canadian physician who was a founder of Johns Hopkins Hospital (and who coincidentally died during the influenza epidemic), called pneumonia "the old man's friend."

Huh? *Friend?* His idea was that the lung condition so common among seniors brought a quicker death and end to suffering. Even today, with pneumonia vaccines available, some doctors who work with the elderly question the wisdom of preventing or aggressively treating pneumonia in patients who are clearly dying, as it only gives the underlying illnesses, such as cancer or heart disease, more time to miserably progress. For more on the ethical considerations of this argument, see "If Pneumonia is the 'Old Man's Friend,' Should it be Prevented by Vaccination? An Ethical Analysis, by Richard Kent Zimmerman. (31)

The word pneumonia is a descriptive term for inflammation of the tiny air sacs in the lungs (alveoli) where oxygen/carbon dioxide exchange takes place, and can have a host of causes, usually infection by either bacteria or virus (or rarely even fungi or parasites), which are most opportunistic when the lungs and immune system are already weak. Vaccines only protect against the viral type.

If your immune system isn't vigorous, the wee beastie microorganisms will use any avenue they can to attack, and being on a ventilator or having a feeding tube opens a clear pathway for them. Seniors may have a difficult time swallowing and often get choked, breathing food or liquids or even saliva into their lungs, resulting in aspiration pneumonia. The risk increases for those who lack mobility and are horizontal while eating or drinking. It is the second leading cause of adult hospitalizations after childbirth, and patients can get it while in the hospital for something else. The mortality rate for patients 85 or over is almost 30%, according to the NIH. It can be a painful "fish out of water" way to go. You work so hard at getting air into your lungs that you are exhausted, yet it does no good once it's there.

Smoking and COPD (Chronic Obstructive Pulmonary Disease, a term that includes both emphysema and chronic bronchitis) increase your susceptibility to pneumonia. If you have been a smoker, you will probably have some degree of COPD, and that is the most common cause. If you have not been a smoker, though, you still can't rule it out, because other environmental factors such as air pollution can cause it as well. I have never been a smoker but do have a mild form of it myself, most likely from growing up in a home heated by a coal stove and tending a wood burner, as well as doing woodworking later in life.

Sleep apnea, or start/stop breathing while sleeping, is more serious than just ticking off your partner with your snoring. It deprives your brain, heart, and all the rest of oxygen, and it is likely to increase with age. Since apnea interrupts deep sleep, it leads to fatigue and can hasten cognitive impairment. It goes hand in hand with being overweight, like Type 2 diabetes. No one likes the thought of a humming, wheezing mask on your face while trying to sleep, but there may be other options. Untreated, it is serious. Losing weight and not over drinking are obvious strategies. If they don't work, it may call for intervention.

Muscle and bone

I first thought to simply label this section "Joints," but I don't want anyone to confuse it with our topic in Chapter 3. Isn't it ironic that a similar-sounding moan coming from the bedroom of a 20-something and of a 70-something is interpreted so differently? One may denote extasy, but the other routine while trying to get out of bed. And how, if male, the meaning of *waking up stiff* is altered so dramatically by the years?

A little joint anatomy: Joints are where bones meet and move against one another. To aid this, most surfaces have a slick lining called a *synovial membrane* further lubricated by synovial fluid, all contained in the somewhat thicker synovial capsule. Ligaments hold bones to bones, so they don't fly apart from one another, and tendons attach muscles to the bones to move them. Neither have a very good blood supply, meaning they don't heal very quickly when injured.

Like anything else that moves against another thing (brake pads on your car, for example), the surfaces eventually wear thin, and you have arthritis. There are lots of different kinds, but this most common "wear and tear" type is *osteoarthritis* and most of us will have it to some degree. If advanced, the lining has disintegrated, and the resulting bone-on-bone movement is very painful. *Rheumatoid arthritis* is an autoimmune disease in which your body goes haywire and begins to attack its own joints, causing pain and inflammation. *Gout*, once the painful sign of an affluent life and excruciatingly painful, most often occurs in the big toe and is caused by a buildup of sharp crystals of uric acid. *Psoriatic arthritis* is similar to rheumatoid arthritis but associated with the skin disease psoriasis.

Even without the pain and swelling of arthritis, the general wearing and drying out of our tendons and ligaments and joints leads to stiffness. Think about the last time you sat in the floor to wrap Christmas presents, and why you now use a table or bed. There are lots of treatments, including anti-inflammatory drugs such as acetaminophen (Tylenol) and NSAIDs like aspirin and ibuprofen (Aleve and Motrin are popular brands). In severe cases, opioids are prescribed for short times, but beware the risk of dependance. Corticosteroid shots directly into the joint (shudder) can be helpful.

Those treatments can be life-changing and make up a multi-billion-dollar industry. The one that is often most effective, though, is free! But it's also hard: *lose weight, and exercise.* Every pound you lose reduces pressure on your knee joint (the one replaced most often) by four pounds. From gout to inflammation, every symptom of osteoarthritis can be mitigated to some degree by maintaining proper weight and a combination of strength and flexibility exercises.

Bursitis and *tendonitis* are more often caused by repetitive strain or injury at any age, but getting older doesn't help, especially for those who are generally out of shape and then "overdo it."

The most mysterious member of the body pain club is *fibromyalgia*. We don't fully know what causes it, and the word itself (from the Latin for "fibrous tissue and muscle pain") is more of a description of symptoms rather than of origin. It can manifest as pain and tenderness throughout the body, fatigue, and sleep disorders. Research indicates that, for some, the disease may be caused by the sufferer's hypersensitivity to the routine pain most of us are able to subconsciously ignore. There could also be genetic factors involved. We simply aren't sure. More women get it than men, and it often begins in middle age, but it is not inflammatory like arthritis. Treatments often include pain relievers and antidepressants. Sometimes anti-seizure medications help block the pain. The condition is made even more frustrating by its lack of focus, sometimes described as "just hurting all over."

Digestion

Back when computer science was relatively new, professors glibly talked about the "GIGO - Garbage In, Garbage Out" axiom. While simplistic, it also explains a lot about our digestive tract, especially as we age. Like the rest of our muscles, our digestive system may not contract as vigorously as it once did, slowing down food and waste. Absorption of nutrients by the intestines may also suffer. Many medications can further inhibit the digestive process, causing constipation. Ulcers that have been silently brewing for years come into their own, and stomach acids may begin to backup into the esophagus, causing heartburn or even GERD (*Gastroesophageal reflux disease*).

All these things can negatively affect your quality of life. If you are constipated you don't feel like going anywhere, and if you have diarrhea you are *afraid* to go anywhere. The number of medications (and their television commercials) available for digestive issues are an indication how widespread the problems are, even among non-seniors.

While you may not be able to avoid all digestive maladies, what you can do is beginning to sound like a broken record: Eat and drink right and get plenty of exercise.

Lots of people are chronically dehydrated because they don't drink enough water and consume too much caffeine. Add diuretics to the mix and the risk increases. Our sensations, such as thirst, may even dull with age and our ability to process sodium, which affects thirst and fluid metabolism, often changes. The solution is simple: drink more fluids. Aim for almost a gallon a day for men and three quarts for women, and do not count caffeinated beverages. Depending on what you eat (particularly fresh fruits and vegetables), food can provide about a fifth of that total. Measure water out in a refrigerator pitcher in the morning if you have trouble keeping track, and maybe add some lemon slices to keep it interesting.

Another common digestive deficit is fiber. This indigestible plant material is mostly devoid of nutrients but carries away waste and can even help prevent diabetes and heart disease. The very best type comes from eating fresh vegetables, fruits, dried legumes, nuts, and whole grains. Fiber supplements make up a 30+ billion dollar a year industry in the United States. They may be needed, but I can't help wondering how much better off we might be if our required intake (shoot for 20-30 grams a day) came from nutrient-rich foods instead of gritty powder.

Your gut microbiome is vitally important but less often addressed. Never feel alone, because your gut is home to trillions of microorganisms, including more than a thousand species of bacteria plus viruses, fungi, and parasites. They help break down food into nutrients that can be absorbed and provide enzymes that allow us to use the B vitamins. They process bile so it can be recycled. They play an important role in the production of necessary fatty acids as well. Aside from all that, our friendly gut microorganisms are the frontline of defense against harmful ones.

How do we keep it healthy? An out-of-balance biome causes problems. Take a powerful antibiotic and it can sometimes give you diarrhea or constipation, right? That's because many of our "good bacteria" get killed off, along with the bad bugs the drug is meant to kill. The same recommendation above concerning high-fiber foods, especially raw vegetables, and whole grains, also provides the conditions for gut health. It can get an extra boost from fermented foods, like sauerkraut and other pickled vegetables and live active culture yogurt. Eat up!

The Senses

Some of us have had sensory deficits our entire lives. I have worn "Coke-bottle" glasses since fourth grade, and multiple ear infections as a youth paired with insufficient hearing protection over my lifetime (including time spent as an adolescent male during the 1970s when rock music was, without debate, *most excellent)* has led to a degree of hearing loss. I travel frequently, and failing vision and hearing are becoming more of a concern while doing so. Changes are often so gradual that we may not even notice. All our senses are likely to lessen as we age, with progression often accelerating around age 50.

Vision: Our eyes have many moving parts involved in seeing detail clearly, and they become less flexible over the years. *Presbyopia,* a natural consequence of aging, is the gradual loss of your ability to focus. It's annoying, and the reason I must take my glasses off and bring an object right up to the end of my nose to do close-up work. Retina cells don't generally regenerate, and the jelly-like "humors" *(aqueous* in front of the lens and *vitreous* between the lens and retina) become cloud. We are all likely to develop "floaters," little clumps of collagen fibers that dance around inside your eye and look like strings or cobwebs or bubbles, jumping away when you try to focus on them. If you see a sudden onset of new floaters, flashes of light, black or blurry spots in your field of vision, see an eye specialist as soon as possible. If the cause is a detached retina, quick treatment can help save your vision.

One of the greatest vision robbers is *age-related macular degeneration,* or AMD. The center focus area of the retina deteriorates so you can only see a side vision view, losing detail. About 80% of cases are "dry AMD," which is gradual. In the less common and more severe "wet AMD," abnormal blood vessels grow under the retina and leak blood and fluid, causing a large blind spot where your center focus should be. *Glaucoma* is another risk because it damages the optic nerve and is usually caused by high fluid pressure in the eye. The dreaded "puff of air" in your ophthalmologist's office tests for glaucoma.

Cataracts are cloudy areas in the lens, keeping light from passing through to focus on the retina. Poor night vision, seeing "halos" around lights, needing brighter lights for work and reading are symptoms. About a fifth of people develop them by age 75. The most common type of cataract surgery involves making a small incision in the eye, breaking up the cataract with ultrasound, fishing them out, and replacing the damaged area with a synthetic intraocular lens, or IOL. In some cases, a laser instead of ultrasound is used to remove the cataract. You may even have a choice, in consultation with your doctor, as to what type of IOL is implanted. Many people choose the new lens to be set for distance, and still wear reading glasses. Some go with the "one eye distance, the other close up" option.

Since most of these eye disorders are so gradual, they are often not diagnosed until they are harder to treat. Even if your vision is acceptable, a regular eye exam is a good idea. There are specific eye health supplements that could be helpful; discuss them with your doctor.

Most of all, if you have diabetes or high blood pressure, keep them controlled and don't smoke. All of these are major risk factors.

Hearing: Your eardrum is yet another piece of tissue that becomes less flexible with age. Take a ticket and get in line, eardrum! Having been around loud noise without adequate hearing protection throughout one's lifetime may hasten onset. Like vision loss, becoming hard of hearing is so gradual that it is often denied. A simple hearing test tells the tale. In severe cases, cochlear implants are used, but for most of us a hearing aid is more likely the answer.

It's amazing how small they are today, a far cry from the deck-of-cards-sized device my grandfather carried in his shirt pocket with a thin red-and-white braided cord trailing up to the earpiece.

Don't be vain. Be evaluated if you notice yourself:

- Asking others to repeat themselves, or just agreeing or nodding when someone is talking even though you aren't completely sure what was said.
- Saying, "Huh?" or "What?" frequently.
- Having activated the Closed Captioning option on your television, even though you tell yourself you don't really need it.
- Being annoyed when someone else mentions how loud your television or stereo is set.
- Having difficulty hearing speech when there is a lot of background noise, such as in an airport.
- Complaining that other people mumble.
- Failing to hear high-pitched sounds, such as car or appliance noises, when asked "Do you hear that sound?"

Hearing evaluations are usually covered under Medicare Part B. While practically unnoticeable by others, hearing aids do take some getting used to, mainly because you have become so accustomed to your hearing loss that they make normal ranges sound too loud. There are probably thousands of sets safely tucked away in drawers across the country after being used only a few days. I know my late father's were! That represents millions of dollars' worth of high-tech equipment wasted because they can be shockingly expensive. Check your insurance and discount plans that may be available through organizations such as AARP, your union, Lions Club, Civitan, or any others with which you have membership. The markup on hearing aids is high, so after other options have been employed, think of the process like buying a car and attempt to negotiate. Nothing ventured, nothing gained.

The hearing aid industry doesn't like this, but in 2022 the FDA established guidelines for an allowable class of Over the Counter (OTC) hearing aids. The maximum amplification is 111 decibels, the deepest ear canal penetration remains at least 10 millimeters from the eardrum, and they must also be volume adjustable.

Now you can self-fit a hearing aid just like you can reading glasses at the drugstore. In fact, that big box store from which you buy 6-packs of romaine lettuce and pick up a big pizza cheap is now one of the leading hearing aid retailers in the country. Name brands can even be purchased online, with a window to return them if they don't work for you. Buyer beware (as with everything else in the world), but the OTC hearing aid option can bring you the very same devices for a lot less money. You decide "Yes, this helps me hear, it feels okay, and I will use it," instead of someone else making that determination for you. I am not downplaying the expertise of hearing aid professionals, but, especially with mild hearing loss, we might do just as well trying simpler models out for ourselves.

Research seems to confirm that choice. A randomized clinical trial conducted by Drs. Karina De Sousa, Vinaya Manchaiah, David Moore, et al (32) found that "a self-fitting OTC hearing aid may be an effective intervention option for individuals with mild to moderate hearing loss and produce self-perceived and clinical outcomes similar to those of an audiologist-fitted hearing aid." Make your own decision, but I know what I am going to try first, and, unfortunately, it won't be long.

Another common hearing issue as we age is tinnitus (I never can figure out which syllable is accented in that pesky word), a high-pitched buzzing, ringing, or roaring sound only you hear. I am all too familiar with it. My own began suddenly in my right ear several years ago and is ever present. Up to a quarter of adults have some degree of tinnitus, and I doubt any of them appreciate it.

Sometimes tinnitus has an identifiable cause, such as an earwax buildup or high doses of some medications, such as NSAIDs. Since these may be remedied, you should consult your doctor if tinnitus develops. More often it is a nerve issue rather than a problem with the eardrum or the tiny bones in the middle ear. Remember the terms *hammer, anvil, stirrup*, and *cochlea* from sixth grade? I seem to remember us boys snickering at that last one, for some reason.

Available treatment options may not seem all that satisfying. Sometimes counseling around how to better live with it helps. Because the sound seems much louder when there is little ambient noise, we often focus on having some other sound to mask it, or at least keep us from concentrating on it, and there are specific sound generating earpieces and bedside machines to produce a soft, pleasant background. Mine seldom bothers me except in the quiet of the night, when trying to fall asleep, and I have devised my own strategy. My wife was perplexed and befuddled when she saw me thread a set of earbuds connected to the bedstand radio into my pillowcase the first night we slept together. (Why, our wedding night, of course!) But falling asleep to the somnolent voices of BBC newsreaders masking that infernal buzz works for me. If I awaken before time to get up, I move my head around on the pillow until I find the earbud and begin listening again.

Research continues, and new treatments may be on the way. With so many sufferers, there certainly is a market, and that's what drives innovation in our society.

We can adjust to hearing and vision loss, and there are tools to help us do so, but there is an important secondary risk. If we have trouble seeing and hearing, we may do fewer things and have contact with fewer people, causing social isolation. Fewer conversations can mean less cognitive challenge, leading to mental decline. People often unintentionally ignore someone with vision and hearing difficulties, other than saying hello and goodbye. Don't settle, and don't just accept, because there are options.

Taste and Smell: I have heard older folks say, "nothing tastes as good as it used to," and they may not be just making it up. If deadened, these closely related senses can lead to loss of appetite and overall enjoyment of one's life. Medications, gum disease, and COVID can all affect your sense of taste, but mostly our salivary glands and our taste buds (sensory cells in the mouth) just stop working as well. Quite a bit of the experience we register as taste is often actually smell, and the same thing applies. Those olfactory sensors grow old and tired, though medications, allergies, and viruses can also affect them. Ask your doctor to check if there is anything causing taste and smell loss, and how it can be remedied. It it's from aging only, it may be time to add two tablespoons of Old Bay Seasoning instead of one.

Touch: The same steady decline applies. Seniors might not

even sense and react to temperature as quickly, putting them more at risk for kitchen and shower burns.

There is yet another risk: Apparently, humans need physical contact with others…to be touched, skin-to-skin. The negative consequences of babies seldom being held is well known, but elder adult touch deficit can also be dire. Called *touch starvation*, it stressed the body, causing production of the stress hormone cortisol, with some effects similar to those of adrenaline. When stress is chronic and cortisol levels don't decrease after the perceived threat has passed, all kinds of bad things can happen over time, including anxiety, depression, digestive problems, memory and concentration decline, sleep problems, heart disease, weight gain, and just about a you-name-it list of things you want to avoid.

When we are touched, oxytocin, dubbed the love hormone, is produced by the hypothalamus, and it has the opposite effect as cortisol.

Why does it happen? Some elderly people have lost their partners, either through death or separation, or physical attraction has waned. A less enlightened generation may still view being "touchy-feely" with negatively, especially men. Younger family members may not touch their older loved ones as much because they perceive them as frail and don't want to inadvertently cause harm. Many of us are natural introverts who were seldom hugged as children, have always been uncomfortable with touch, and it's catching up with us. *-slowly raises hand-*

We are not too old to change. Come here, you!

Cognitive decline: If you think your memory is just as good as it was when you were younger, you are probably just not remembering how good it was.

People joke about it, but it's not funny. I go down to the garage to bring up a case of water and come back upstairs without it. I miss a turnoff on a route I have driven a thousand times. Then I begin to doubt myself on other things. I know I paid the bills this month…or did I? Two months ago, I got a past due notice on the utility bill, for the first time in my entire life! I am getting leery of traveling on my own, even. – Female

I hate it too. While we admire geezers still described as sharp as a tack, most everyone will suffer some degree of cognitive decline, including memory loss (the most common), difficulty concentrating and making decisions, and getting confused about directions. If severe enough, it can affect our ability to live independently, and even mild cases can lead to frustration, isolation, and depression. It may be inevitable; like every other part of the body, the brain is likely to experience some degree of decline with age. It's expected and probably unavoidable if you live long enough; almost a quarter of us have mild cognitive impairment by age 65, according to the Columbia University Irving Medical Center.

You should still talk with your doctor about it, though, because there are many other factors that can affect it, such as medications and blood chemistry imbalances, and adjusting these things may help.

Two dreaded terms describing more severe cognitive decline are *dementia* and *Alzheimer's disease.* The difference is sometimes confusing, but, unlike mild and expected cognitive impairment, they are serious disorders and not inevitable effects of aging. Only 3% of those between 65 and 69 have dementia, rising to 35% in our 90s. (33)

Dementia is not a specific disease, but instead a general term for cognitive decline symptoms. Alzheimer's disease is a specific type (and the most common, among several) of dementia that is progressive and may affect one side of the brain first instead of the whole. If it affects the left side language goes first, and the right, visual and spatial relationships. As opposed to vascular dementia which occurs due impaired blood flow (such as in strokes), Alzheimer's fills the brain up with plaques that disrupt brain signals. As those connections wither, the entire brain may begin to shrink, and when it advances, lack of brain function can lead to death. There is no cure. While new medicines and treatments are in the works (always), the best we can sometimes do is help the sufferer be as safe and healthy as possible while supporting his or her family and caregivers.

Most of us have heard the horror stories about a kind and gentle person becoming aggressive and dangerous, not knowing spouses or children, or wondering off and getting lost. Those aren't exaggerations. Three issues:

-When to seek help: If you ask the same questions repeatedly, get lost, stop attending to routine hygiene and duties, or are not able to identify family and friends, talk to your doctor. You don't have to assume the worst just because you become forgetful. Leaving a pot on the stove for so long it boils over is dangerous, but one instance of doing it doesn't necessarily mean something serious is going on with your brain.

-Manage risk factors: An important one you can't do anything about is your genetics. Having a family history of dementia increases (but does not guarantee) your own likelihood of getting it. But there are many things you can control. Smoking and drinking too much are significant risk factors, as are atherosclerosis, hypertension, obesity, diabetes, and high cholesterol. Now, don't see this as a green light, but there is some evidence that complete abstinence from alcohol consumption may also not be helpful.

-Keep your mind and body active. Mental activities that challenge the brain are essential. "Use it or lose it" applies to it just as much as to muscle tone. Stay socially engaged, work puzzles, read thought-provoking books (like this one!), learn new skills, travel, have involved conversations. Provided you don't smoke, and maybe even if you are just now quitting, the number one thing you can do to reduce your risk of dementia is to *keep moving*. According to a combined analysis of 16 correlational studies by the Alzheimer's Society UK, regular exercise can reduce your risk of dementia by about 28%, and of Alzheimer's disease specifically by 45%. You can't find much better odds than those.

SO, NOW WHAT?

What a litany of things that can, and likely will, go wrong!

I hate going to the doctor. They just want to keep bringing you back to make money, and they hardly look at you but keep prescribing more medicine. -Male

Seniors often put off going to the doctor because we don't want to hear what they say. We don't want to be told we need to exercise and lose weight. We lie to them about how much we drink. There are many illnesses that were fatal a couple of generations ago but today are commonly cured, though, and they may have few symptoms until it's too late. Seniors should have regular bloodwork and other diagnostic exams. Unless you notice some kind of change or you know you have a condition needing attention, an annual checkup might be sufficient. Past that, it is perfectly acceptable to question your doctor when things like sleep studies or full body scans are suggested. I am not saying you should refuse them out of hand, but ask questions to make sure you understand the risks and potential benefits and make up your own mind. Be willing to seek a second opinion if you have doubts.

Beware medication creep. It seems like doctors are more willing to add medications than remove them even if their continued benefit is negligible, resulting in so many pills you may not feel like eating breakfast after swallowing all your morning doses. Insist on a medication review at least annually, going over each medicine, what it is doing for you, and whether it can be reduced or eliminated. If you see more than one doctor, make sure each knows all that you are taking.

What about all those pills in advertising targeted at seniors? There seems to be supplements for everything, and happy, sincere-sounding elders in beautiful settings are eager to tell us about their benefits. That's the importance of annual bloodwork. If you have a vitamin or mineral deficiency, you may need to supplement those things. If you don't, their usefulness is debatable, and your doctor should be on that debate team. Many supplements may do no harm (to anything but your pocketbook) but evaluating the good they do may be illusive. "I feel better while taking it" might be enough for you, though.

I am a science-y guy and something needs to show me evidence before I sign on. In today's information free-for-all, it is possible to access valid information from reliable sources, and that's the key. Look at the NIH, CDC, Mayo Clinic, JAMA, Harvard, Cleveland Clinic, Heart Association, Lung Association, Cancer

Society, and well-known research names you can trust. They will not have all the answers and there may be gray area recommendations, but medicine is still at the intersection of science and art. Double-blind placebo-controlled studies repeated over and over with similar results are the standard. In such studies, red yeast rice extract has been shown to lower cholesterol in some people, apple cider vinegar has been shown to lower blood sugar in others, and meditation has been shown to lower blood pressure for selected folks. Will they work for you? I can't answer that, but consultation with your doctor is a good place to start.

So much stuff. Where does it all end? We know where it ends. Pay attention and do what you can do while you still can.

THE TAKEAWAY

Eat a healthy diet (something close to the Mediterranean diet is often viewed as one of the best, but your choices need to be sustainable, and many seniors don't get sufficient healthy plant and dairy and lean protein), don't smoke or over drink, get enough sleep and plenty of exercise, stay mentally and socially involved, and have regular medical checkups. Rocket science, right?

You already know every bit of that but change and self-discipline are tough. If you want to narrow it down to what to do first, what to do *immediately*, here it is: Get up and get moving. Make walking and other exercise as much a part of your life as brushing your teeth. Start substituting fresh (and some raw) vegetables for processed foods and add whole grains. Stop watching so much television and staring at other screens. Get out and do more things with actual (as opposed to virtual) people. You heard it here first, folks.

5 THE HEARSE AND THE U-HAUL

You're going to die, and it will probably be sooner than it has been. But there are things you can do to make the time you have left better.

"How much would you like to leave behind?" an annoying insurance/investment agent once asked me at my dining room table. "All of it," was my quick reply. "I might as well want that, because that's exactly what's going to happen." In the words of the late Charlie Kuhn (my father), "I ain't seen a hearse with a U-Haul behind it yet." Dad could be pithy. He also said, paraphrasing someone else I'm sure, "If someone says 'It ain't the money, it's the principle of the thing,' it's really the money." I have yet to see him proven wrong.

Stories about family members feeling slighted by not receiving something to which they felt entitled are almost universal. I have seen sibling and cousin and step-relative relationships irreparably damaged after a decedent's (the legal term for a dead person...work that into conversation today!) estate has been distributed. My nonscientific theory is that most of those folks were looking for something to break up over, and not getting grandma's outdoor flowerpot just gave them an excuse.

But before you leave it all behind, you must have some of it in the first place. You have worked hard in life and believe you are entitled to a long, comfortable retirement without deprivation. Most of us, though, do not draw as much money in retirement as we did while working, just when we have more time to spend it on things we want to do. We supplement it by withdrawing from savings and investments that may not continue to grow as fast as we deplete them. If only we knew our expiration date, we could calculate how much to spend, right? We could enjoy it down to the very end, dropping our last quarter into a gumball machine a minute before the heavenly alarm went off.

For many people, senior or non, life is a paycheck-to-paycheck proposition, but perhaps you have considerable resources and experience dealing with investments. Money decisions are important and can be complicated, so we often need advice, and it can be like "Daniel walking into the Lion$' Den." I am sure most are skilled and ethical, and if you have substantial assets, you can probably get a free lunch at Applebee's to hear their pitch. Here's a word to remember: *fiduciary,* someone who has a legal duty to act in the best financial interest of someone else. If you use a financial advisor to manage your money, I suggest making sure she or he is one. Ask, and make sure the answer is firm, instead of something fuzzy like, "Oh, yes, I *can* act as a fiduciary. Have you had that Sizzlin' Butter Pecan Blondie?"

They do not provide this service for free, of course. They may charge a flat fee, or an annual percentage of your assets. With the ease of investing today (both a blessing and a curse?), it is perfectly acceptable to pay a financial advisor for consultation and then do it yourself instead of turning your money over for her to manage. Remember that, just because an advisor is a fiduciary does not mean she or he is good at the job. "Yes, it is my responsibility to act in your best interest, but I also really suck at it" still gets you nowhere but the poorhouse.

Where to begin? A good place that will not take a cent from you (but also will not buy you lunch, unfortunately) is the Consumer Financial Protection Bureau, an official government agency. Their website (www.consumerfinance.gov) is an incredible resource, especially under the heading *Tools for Financial Security in Later*

Life. There are videos and downloadable guides on just about every topic you can imagine, from early retirement planning to Social Security to Reverse Mortgages (that's how Tom Selleck is able to drive such nice cars, right?)

At the risk of raising ire: for some, it seems like the main objective of financial planning is to avoid one's estate going for nursing home care, and I get it. We want the money we worked and scrimped and saved for to go to our family, not to Genesis HealthCare ($5.70 billion annual revenue), Life Care Centers of America ($4.30 billion annual revenue) or the Ensign Group ($3.025 annual revenue). What, you thought all those nursing homes were small local businesses, in an industry with a 3.32% projected growth rate? (34)

We are great at getting people to live longer. What they are to do with those years, and we as a society do *with* those seniors, is another story.

Medicare does not pay for nursing home care except for relatively short stays as part of rehabilitation. As a rule, patients pay for it until their money is gone, and then the Medicaid program picks up the bill. The monthly cost averages between $8,000 and $9,000 a month. Maybe your 401(k) produces that. Mine (ahem) does not. I can't make many general statements past that because Medicaid programs vary from state to state.

My parents worked hard their whole lives. They didn't have much, but wanted what little they did have to go to their family. But after my father died, my mother ended up in a nursing home, and every cent was gone in less than a year, even with her whole Social Security check and little pension going toward her care. Now she gets to keep $35 a month. It's called a "personal needs allowance,' and it's supposed to cover clothes, getting her hair done, and everything else. I really don't care that there's nothing left for us when she dies, but did she really deserve to lose everything because she couldn't take care of herself anymore? It's pitiful, really. - Female

Yes, so it is. I know from personal experience. It's a national issue that will just get more problematic as we Baby Boomers transition from embarrassing golfcart parades in The Villages to complaining *Not oatmeal again?* in the Serenity Meadows Personal Care Center. A rather unpopular view, though, is what better use is there for my own money than to make sure I am being cared for properly, until that runs out and the taxpayers must do it? Isn't that how it *should* be used?

What's the answer? I am afraid I haven't got it. My great-grandmother, whose dad was a Confederate soldier, lived with my grandparents when I was a lad. (I was her favorite, by the way, no matter what my many cousins say) That's what families did back then. Here in the United States, nursing home care is viewed as institutionalization, whereas in much of Western Europe it is considered a "community-based residential service." Words matter. And over there it is usually funded through taxes or through *subsidized* long-term care insurance without the requirement that the resident become destitute first.

We have our priorities, don't we?

I am not a fiduciary, since I would prefer you buy this book instead of reading it for free at Barnes and Noble, but I think the following advice is in your best interest:

Figure out exactly what you want. What brings you joy? Use the "better, rather than more" standard. The Burmeisters from church might brag about going on five cruises a year (good for them!), but would that bring *you* joy? Budget out how to do the best of what you love, what you look forward to, and incorporate more of it in little, inexpensive doses in your everyday life. Hold that thought; in Chapter 7, we will talk about never turning down the good because it isn't perfect and dropping the façade of affluence (even if you are, indeed, affluent).

Don't forget taxes (as if they would let you) and the potential future of Social Security. When I received my first retirement estimate form Uncle Sam, I thought *Woo hoo! I can live on that!* And I do. But that was a *before tax* estimate, and the reality is markedly different. Your financial advisor may have suggestions about how to legitimately pay less in taxes, but you aren't going to avoid them unless you are so rich you wouldn't notice paying them anyhow. Those are the folks who are able to, somehow.

When to take Social Security is another issue without definitive answer because you don't know your expiration date. Most advice I have read suggests waiting until your full retirement age (usually around 67 for most of us, depending on birth year) if you are in reasonably good health, and your monthly benefit even increases the longer you wait after that up until age 70. But the whole thing is based on average lifespan. Take it earlier, and you draw it longer. Wait and you draw more per month, but for a shorter amount of time. Which causes you to end up with more in the long run depends on when your alarm goes off, so the decision must be made without full data. Don't you hate that? If you have other substantial income, your Social Security may be federally taxed (remember that when looking at your estimates…gee, thanks, Ronnie. Would the orphaned but fun-loving Drake McHugh have done that in Kings Row? Maybe.) and even taxed again by the state, depending on which one you call home.

Great Expectations is one of the world's finest novels, but it's not your story. If your family thinks you are becoming a big, ah, *Dickensian* because you are less generous to them as they progress in life, so be it. Are you picking up the check every time you are out with your family? Paying for vacations so they will spend time with you? Funding grandchildren's education? The "give it to them now while I can see them enjoy it" philosophy may be valid if you are well set and it brings you joy, but honesty evaluate if it has become an expectation, great or otherwise.

There are more fun things to be obsessed over. For some seniors, *my money and my stuff* and *will I have enough* and *what will happen to it when I die* seems to be all they can think about, and every conversation comes around to it. Well, friends, we have already answered the last part of that question for you unequivocally: you will leave it behind. All of it. Do your due diligence to make sure it all goes where you want it to go and leave it at that, because *you can't control anything after you die.* Each minute obsessing over it is a minute spent not laughing or learning or living (or Chapter 1-ing). Sometimes the obsession comes in the form of trying to make sure everything you leave is distributed with precise equality down to the penny, and decisions are made in an attempt to please everyone else rather than your own wishes. There may be legal requirements concerning spousal property, but you are under no obligation to leave "exactly the same," for example, to a child you have greatly subsidized as an adult versus one who has been fiercely independent. Unless it brings you joy! In that case, do it, but not just because someone might get pouty at your post-mortem self. Have a will and keep it updated. I don't care how much or how little you leave, not having a will can cause lots of things you don't want to happen, perhaps with strangers making the decisions. "What do I care? I'll be dead!" you say. Valid point. Consider it an act of self-reflection, deciding what (and who) is important to you. There are "will kits" out there, and some may be sufficient for your needs, especially personalized forms from one of the reputable online services. State laws vary, so using the fill-in-the-blank the form in the back of the Ladies Aid Society Cookbook is probably not a good idea.

Like working on your own car these days, it could be the case that you need a professional in order to keep from doing more harm than good. Yes, it will cost you a few bucks. A simple will may be under $300, with more complex scenarios costing more. For example, setting up a trust is sometimes the instrument most likely to produce your desired result, and that will be pricier. Get estimates for the best deal, but this isn't the place to cheap out.

Remember that you do not have to leave everything to family. Sometime friends are just as close, and charities that you believe in and supported in life will appreciate being remembered. Appointing an executor is not a popularity contest, or the right of the firstborn. Choose someone with bureaucratic abilities and you trust to be honest in carrying out your wishes. While we love those dramatic will-reading scenes in movies (my favorite is in *Knives Out* with Daniel Craig), there may not be any good reason to keep the contents of your will secret from your descendants. Discussing it beforehand can help everyone understand your wishes and avoid conflict. But discuss it and then drop it.

Pre-planning (and pre-paying) your funeral/body disposition

arrangements is a great gift to those you are leaving behind. If you have ever had to unexpectedly attend to these duties for a deceased loved one as I have, you know what I mean. Inform your family, show them the paperwork, and then once again drop it. Make sure you have all the necessary Advance Medical Directives in place (more on that later).

THE TAKEAWAY

You came in without a cent. You're going out the same way, except for that one coin necessary to pay Charon the boatman for passage. What you work for and accumulate in between has been guided (even dictated) by necessity and expectation and identity. Now is your chance for it to be guided by the joy it brings you, not someone else's expectations.

6 GET ON MY LAWN

You're going to die, and it will probably be sooner than it has been. But there are things you can do to make the time you have left better.

Oh, great. Now he's getting touch-feely. We're all supposed to love one another, right? Well, that's just not me. Never has been. I'm fine, thanks. I am happier keeping to myself, and don't really need anybody. -Male

Yeah. That's me.

How do we know about the importance of relationships as we age? It's not like there have been long-term studies, since this is a new-age-y kind of thing, right?

Contraire. One of the most important "For further reading" recommendations I can make is *Aging Well: Surprising Guideposts to a Happier Life from the Landmark Study of Adult Development* by George E. Vaillant (Little, Brown Spark, December 2008) and *Triumphs of Experience* by the same author (Belknap Press, 2012). Harvard Medical School began following 824 teenage subjects, some rich and some poor, back in the late 1930s. A couple notable rich ones were Ben Bradlee (later editor of the Washington Post) and a young scion of a Boston political family named John F. Kennedy. These subjects have been tracked, examined, and interviewed ever since. Today the study continues with their descendants and new participants, now numbering more than 1,000.

And what does eight decades of research show? Lots of things, obviously, but Dr. Vaillant himself sums up the main conclusion, that warm relationships are the single greatest factor in living a satisfying life, like this: *Happiness is love. People with good relationships, regardless of social background, are healthier, more productive, more financially successful, live longer, and pass more positives along to their children.*

Read the books. They are astounding and cover almost every aspect of living and aging in America.

(By the way, the study found that aging liberals have more sex, remaining sexually active into their 80s, while conservative men ceased sexual relations at an average age of 68. Some of you bros might want to consider buying a different color ball cap.)

When I consider the importance of my relationships with my own daughters and stepson, it's incomprehensible when I hear of other parents who no longer have contact with their adult children and other family members. Something happened that made them all mad at one another. They moved away and just drifted apart. They no longer have anything in common with one another. They were from a first marriage and now have different family dynamics. It's sad and most often avoidable.

All those things can apply equally to friends who aren't family as well. We are suffering an epidemic of loneliness, and it is literally killing us. Surgeon General Dr. Vivek Murthy told *USA TODAY* in December 2003, "Most of us probably think of loneliness as just a bad feeling. It turns out that loneliness has far greater implications for our health when we struggle with a sense of social disconnection, being lonely or isolated."

The COVID epidemic certainly didn't help. Being stuck at home except for unavoidable and careful expeditions out for food while keeping our distance from others became easier after a time, and then we became complacent with doing the same after the vaccines brought some degree of normalcy back to our lives, but the problem was increasing even before the virus reached our shores.

A study by Harvard (separate from the long-term study

mentioned above) with 950 participants in 2020 showed that about 36% of us feel serious loneliness, which has strong causal relationships with depression, substance abuse, anxiety, and even heart disease. As we age, it is a significant risk factor in developing dementia, stroke, and premature death. While loneliness is subjected and difficult to gauge when self-reported, social isolation is the more easily measured lack of social relationships and contact.

This isn't just about no longer knowing anyone who owns a pickup truck when you have a sofa to move. It's life and death. Have you seen someone's rapid decline after losing a spouse and there was not a significant, lively social network to help counteract the resulting aloneness? It's common. As a health risk, it's finally getting its due. The National Academies of Sciences, Engineering, and Medicine reconfirms that social isolation is associated with, among other things, the onset of heart disease, hypertension, obesity, a weakened immune system, cognitive decline, dementia, and Alzheimer's disease, depression, and early death. Its negative effect can even be compared with smoking vs. not smoking. (35) (see also The Growing Problem of Loneliness, J. T. and S. Cacioppo, *Lancet* 2018; 391 (10119): 426).

Not enough? A committed romantic relationship lowers mortality risk by 49%, and having a strong social network reduces it by 45%, according to a meta-analysis by M. Aaraska. (36)

Failing eyesight, hearing, mobility, and reduced involvement in physically demanding things like sports make things even worse. And today's technology of having 136 channels of instant entertainment on our 72-inch screen plus interacting with "friends" we never see in real life for hours every day via Facebook give the illusion that we are not socially isolated.

The lack of satisfying emotionally intimate relationships is literally killing us. Old friends die or move to Florida, with similar result. We're without a partner, either through death or divorce. The kids and grandkids are all busy with their own lives. *Those women at the senior center look down on me because I was never part of their golf club social circle, and all those old guys down at the K of C hall do is brag and argue with one another over nothing. Who needs them?*

Apparently, you and I do.

When you lose a spouse or close friend or your kids grow up and you are no longer involved in their activities, there are usually concentric rings of other relationships lost as well. As we age, the cumulative effect catches up to us because we often lack both the opportunity and motivation to replace lost friends with new ones.

Long term relationships can die either a natural-but-avoidable death, or be *killed off.* Let me explain:

A relationship's natural-but-avoidable death is usually from neglect and malnourishment. We starve it. No matter how many decades ago a relationship began and how close it once was, it is always begging *what have you done for me lately?* It takes work, just at the stage of life when you believe you shouldn't really have to work at anything anymore. It may also require a financial investment, especially if you are separated by distance.

I lost close relationships during the writing of this book. You have already been introduced to the late Mark Deskins, my walking partner with whom I graduated from high school. We seldom saw one another more than two or three times a year, but were in contact through messages every few days, usually about inconsequential things. We were comfortable and had just as much fun together sitting around the fire pit or in suits speaking conference at the Mayflower Hotel or slogging through boot-sucking bogs in Ireland. The time together seemed so effortless because of the work we put into cultivating it. There was almost always something planned, even if it was in the distant future, like another walk (maybe the Cotswolds this time) or taking our grandsons to Ireland, or something as simple as he and his wife stopping by on their way to Florida for the winter even if it is a bit out of their way.

A few months ago, I received a text from Mark's wife at about 4:00 AM. The evening before, Mark had driven several miles to meet former work colleagues for lunch and came home to a perfectly average evening. Then he had a heart attack and died, at age 64. He was two days younger than me. I still catch myself about to send him a photo or joke or news article.

I couldn't bring myself to attend his memorial service, and feel rather like a coward for it.

My mother died at almost 93, and a friend and writing collaborator who happened to have been one of my students years ago came to the funeral to offer his condolences. Exactly two weeks later, I attended *his* funeral, another victim of a heart attack at only 51 years old.

And then there was that a 19-pound (though she would be *scandalized* for me to broadcast that. She loved snacks, okay? So do I. Don't judge) Cavalier King Charles spaniel named Katie. I did not buy her (my wife did) and I am not a dog person, but she was my constant companion.

Another long-term relationship was feared lost over today's cultural and political tribalism, but we both realized how important it is and pulled back from the abyss.

All of that occurred during the year and a half it took me to research and write the book you are holding. It has kinda sucked.

Three of those three relationships ended due to the intervention of the Grim Reaper. As to the other, there is always enough blame to go around. In such a situation, you may ask yourself *Did I try again, and again, and again to reconnect?* Have I developed new relationships to make up for vacancies? Did we kill off a friendship, or did it die of malnutrition?

So, what do we do? What should *I* do?

THE TAKEAWAY

Make a conscious effort, with specific goals: I am going to meet people, develop new relationships, and strengthen old ones. You don't have to be a creepy stalker who looks needy, but be open to cultivating interactions into something more.

Become a member of new groups and return to groups you have abandoned. Yes, they can be annoying and boring and seem pointless. But if it isn't costing you much more than time that would otherwise be spent in front of some type of screen, you haven't really lost much, now have you? Groups that have regular meetings push you into repeated contact, but don't let yourself get trapped into duties you don't enjoy or feel are worth your time. If a new member joins, be the one who takes the time to get to know her instead of just shaking a hand, saying, "Welcome!" and then ignoring her.

Plan a get together. You don't have to have known someone since 4-H camp to say, "Hey, I'm grilling out Saturday afternoon. Why don't you drop by?" If no one comes (which could happen), try again. After four or five times, maybe it's okay to give up on that person, but give it at least that many. Don't be surprised if there is no reciprocation. It can get irritating to always be the host and never the invitee, I know. Subtle hints can sometimes work. Your soiree doesn't have to be costly or elaborate. One of my few successes after moving to the beach was a simple garage party for St. Patrick's Day with snacks and Irish music. Around 20 folks dropped in and out over a couple of hours. If I hadn't insisted on wearing my Irish National tartan kilt and leading a pub tune singalong, there may have been more.

Be open to conversations in public places. Work on those *Don't' talk to me* nonverbal vibes you are giving off at the bookstore or church or at happy hour. This is tough for me (a natural introvert), but practice makes perfect. If it's not comfortable all the time, choose a day and say, "Only today, I will start up a conversation with someone I don't already know." Then repeat next week.

Consider why old friendships ended and how (and if) they can be resurrected. This may be the hardest of all. Old people get more and more stubborn. Over time, perceived small hurts and slights grow in minds not otherwise occupied. The friend who didn't return your call or come to your birthday party may eventually become responsible for all kind of evils and ills in your mind as you scrutinize your years together.

Plan new activities with family members. Many siblings find themselves only having contact in matters involving their aging parents. We gather on holidays at the parent's insistence and need to cooperate on their healthcare and financial matters. When the parents are gone, so is the contact. I know. We have led independent lives from our family members but have a shared history of both joy and pain. That should account for something more than silence until their grandchildren's graduation announcements go out. Doing the same things year after year out of a feeling of obligation might lose meaning and be easy to jettison. Plan something different together.

And forgive them. Maybe your siblings or cousins or others have treated you poorly in the past. You feel slighted, cheated, ignored, or even bullied. We don't forget (well, sometimes we might. See our discussion of dementia), but we *can* forgive. There is probably a side to the story you haven't considered, and you won't understand it better unless you talk about it. "I have been successful, but you never seem to acknowledge it and always dismiss what I have done and my opinions. I know you're the oldest and I love you, but we're not kids anymore. Can we talk about it?" Your big sister may be floored that you think that way, but your nonthreatening request to deal with your feelings instead of keeping them on slow simmer for the rest of your days might bring you closer than you ever were in the past.

Or let them go. Sad as it is, some long-term relationships are kept alive for no good reason, be they with family or friends. Do what you can to repair them, and that often means initiating difficult conversations. Try. Try again. But if a relationship brings nothing but stress and frustration, let it go, even if it's older than that ragged college sweatshirt you haven't fit into for forty years. The one that brings back all those memories. The one you still love knowing is somewhere in the closet even if you haven't seen it in ages.

Determine to replace it with a new one, one that fits, and I'm not talking about the sweatshirt.

7 OLD RULES

You're going to die, and it will probably be sooner than it has been. But there are things you can do to make the time you have left better.

Since one of the complaints older people have is that they sometimes feel listless, I am giving you a list. Let's call these *"Eight Rules To Keep You From Aging Disgracefully."* After all the reading, research, writing, and living I have done to produce this book, it seems our objective really does boil down to these things. Here they are:

1. Never turn down the good because it isn't perfect.
2. Put real effort into figuring out what is important to you.
3. Push yourself.
4. Stop being a scorekeeper.
5. Focus on relationships and experiences, not stuff.
6. Drop the façade.
7. And the sense of privilege!
8. Live in the real world, not the screen world or the past world.

How can we apply them, right now?

1. NEVER TURN DOWN THE GOOD BECAUSE IT
    ISN'T PERFECT

We all have wants and desires and dreams. We look forward to things and fondly remember good times and visualize what we want to do, to happen, to experience. Most of those will turn out to be great, but not necessarily exactly as we envisioned them, and even many of the things we dread will seem not as bad as we feared when we look back at them later.

What does get even worse as we age, though, is regret over things undone. In her book *The Top Five Regrets of the Dying: A Life Transformed by the Dearly Departing* (37), Bronnie Ware shares her experiences working as a palliative caregiver. Author Daniel H. Pink, in *The Power of Regret: How Looking Backward Moves Us Forward* (38), gives his insight after spending years researching regret. I recommend both books. While there are some differences, they draw the same conclusion: we are much more likely to regret things *undone* than *things we did*. That Hollywood death scene isn't likely to happen. We are not likely to draw loved ones close to hear our final words such as "I wish I hadn't taken those family cruises with y'all" or "Building that cabin in the mountains? Why, oh why, didn't I spend that time at the office instead? Don't make my mistake!"

Too often, that undone list is a result of waiting for things to be perfect. We have the perfect amount of money and the perfect amount of time and can get the perfect room and travel arrangements and weather and group of companions and everything else. Just perfect!

Good luck with that. Did your parents have a *perfect* marriage? Were they *perfect* at parenting? Yet here you are. That $50,000 wedding you paid for? It was such a good time! But it did drizzle for a while, a dozen people sent an RSVP but didn't show despite your still having to pay for their plate at dinner, and Uncle Eugene got a little loud and sloppy during cocktail hour and the marriage only lasted 18 months. Are those the things about it you will recall while sitting in the nursing home someday? Remember, the time will come when your memories of doing things with friends and family will be the most precious things you have. Reducing your store of them because everything must be *just so* for you to do something will likely be one of your biggest regrets.

My cousins get a beach house on Catalina Island for a week every summer and invited us to come join them for a couple of days. It would have been fun, but we would have had to share a bathroom with one of the other couples instead of having one exclusively, so we declined. After all, it's not worth going somewhere if it's not as nice and convenient as our own home. -Female

I always thought I would be able to see the Rolling Stones someday, but they aren't close enough that I wouldn't have to stay in a hotel, and I hate trying to park around a crowded stadium, and tickets close to the stage are pricy, and I really don't like big crowds anymore, and my wife isn't interested in them, and.... -Male

Come on dude. If Mick, Keef, and Ronnie, all almost old enough to be your daddy, are still making the effort, the least you can do is stop being such a wuss and making excuses.

Really want a thirty-foot boat, but can only afford a twenty-footer? Thinking about a steak from Ruth's Chris but your budget strongly suggests Outback? You just watched the train scene with Tom Cruise and Rebecca De Mornay in *Risky Business* (1983) and think it might be fun to recreate it on the Warminster Line between Willow Grove and Glenside but there are lubrication and ED and prying eyes issues? Always dreamed of rolling up to your fiftieth class reunion in a convertible Mercedes just to see the look on Tony Fonatelli's face (but own a Hyundai Sonata) and casually drop into conversation how you rent that house in Tuscany even though we know there are no houses to rent in Tuscany anymore? You want all your children and grandchildren with you for Passover this year, but your daughter's lame husband insists they split the time with HIS dorky family as well, so you can only get part of the crew for part of the holiday?

Well, then! I just won't do any of them at all if I can't do them exactly the way I want!

And you will die with regret. Go to Outback, patiently satisfy your partner and yourself to the extent that it can happen in the seclusion of your own bedroom, detail that Sonata and wish Tony Fonatelli a happy life, save up for a 5-day Trafalgar bus tour of Tuscany, and hide-and-seek the heck out of that Afikomen with whatever kids show up. Chances are good that, in the end, what you remember from any of those things will be positive, no matter if they seemed cut-rate at the time. Opportunities delayed are often opportunities lost. The big hourglass won't get turned again, and enjoying what is obtainable for you today isn't "settling." It's called *living.*

Being a perfectionist, you will always be disappointed and focus on what's missing instead of what's present. It's self-sabotaging, and not pleasant for those around you. Those times when you had a house full of family without quite enough room can create a lot of laughs while waiting for the water heater to refill. How many memories do you make sitting at home because you won't stay at a Super 8 or travel in Economy or experience a concert in the nosebleed section? Because you won't *settle?*

I am no master of this craft. I have always been a rather cautious, responsible guy. But I took my family to Europe on the cheap for the first time when I still had a mortgage, and my daughters were young teens. Yes, it was a Trafalgar bus tour and still stretched my resources. But it was one of the best investments I ever made, because decades later, it still repays me many times over in stories and memories. As an out-of-shape senior citizen, I have hiked in Scotland and Ireland, and ridden the train cross country, Seattle to Philadelphia, in a sleeper compartment simply because I had always wanted to do it.

The scenery through the Rockies is spectacular. I am sure it would have been more fun with a travel companion and I threw out the invitation. When it came time for a commitment, no one wanted to take that much time (they're retired), spend that much money (not that much, done on the cheap, and they all have plenty), just weren't sure they could sleep comfortably on a train, etc. etc. etc. Hm…maybe it was just spending that much time in close quarters with me? That's fair. But failing to do it, even by myself, will not be a nursing home regret for me. Now I need to walk among the sequoias and see the Aurora Borealis and visit the four states I have somehow missed (Alaska, Kansas, and a couple of Dakotas…I am open to invitations!) and several other things.

That's regret over things undone. But can you guess the biggest source of regrets people have about things they DID? It involves what Pink calls "moral regret." You bullied someone. You were an unfaithful lover or friend. You chose selfishness or unkindness or intolerance. Just try forgetting about those wrongs and slights between games of bingo in the nursing home dining room; unless dementia has set in, it might not be so easy. Live in such a way that those things are few, and relatively minor. If you already have a long list of moral regrets, stop doing things that add to it. Remember the Ghost of Marley in that scene from *A Christmas Carol*: "I wear the chain I forged in life," replied the Ghost. "I made it link by link, and yard by yard." You and I are also chain makers, no less than Jacob. It's your choice.

2. PUT REAL EFFORT INTO FIGURING OUT WHAT IS IMPORTANT TO YOU

Rule number 2 is more closely related to rule number 1 than you may think at first. Sometimes choosing to leave things undone and finding perfectionist excuses is caused by not being sure you really want something in the first place and provides an easy way to avoid commitment. Waiting until you are no longer physically able to do important things is not the time to figure out exactly what those things might be.

It sounds easy, doesn't it? You know what you like, dislike, and want to do. But, as the sand runs out and the time you have left to spend becomes dearer, living a life reminiscent of rolling down the highway with your parents, spouse, and kids all in the car and asking "Okay, where do we want to stop to eat?" makes no sense. You don't have that kind of time.

It's strange that we spend so little effort thinking about something so integral to our happiness. Not only do you want to spend your remaining time/financial/mental resources on things that really matter to you today, but you may also need to make decisions about how to leave things to accomplish your goals after you die. In a conversation with financially well-off friends not long ago, we all agreed that it is not our primary objective in waning years to make our children rich when we die. If that happens, great, but we are not depriving ourselves of what we really want in the meantime. They should be self-sufficient, and we worked hard to help them get that way.

On the other hand, I know an older couple with a disabled adult child, and that person's continued welfare after their death is understandably of paramount importance to them, driving many of their life decisions.

The first step is to think about what makes you happy. I hope your list is long. Spending time with friends and family, travel, having a comfortable home, tinkering with crafts and scrapbooks or antiques or woodworking or helping run the parish food pantry or quietly sitting on the beach with a book or fishing or walking your dog or line dancing or working on your 1973 Dodge Dart Swinger with black vinyl top? You may finally start your own business from home, or even continue working at your present job with reduced hours. If it brings you pleasure and is not harmful (some things, such as drinking and gambling, become problematic if done immoderately, of course), then you should concentrate on making it a bigger part of your life.

At any age, though, what we believe will make us happy is dictated by our past experiences and conjecture but still has many unknowns. It's what one of my professors long ago was fond of calling an *epistemological problem*. Sometimes people move to an area they enjoyed as a vacation destination for years but retire there and hate it. You may love being with your children and grandkids, but living next door could bring on a very different dynamic that isn't so cozy after all.

Eddie Samson, a friend and colleague of mine, gives a presentation on retirement he calls *Finding Your Passion*, and it made me think. I will not be judgmental if someone chooses potential decades of senior citizendom intent on just collecting enough of a pension to get by, watching a lot of television, running errands for their kids and grandkids, and waiting for it all to end.

That's their right. But most of us will agree that is exactly what we want to avoid, a purgatory of endless days that seem to go by quickly and slowly at the same time. We need passion. "The mass of men lead lives of quiet desperation," Thoreau wrote in *Civil Disobedience and Other Essays*, unfortunately leaving half the population out of the "mass." Most of us are happier and healthier with objectives, deadlines, things to accomplish and things to look forward to until the time runs out with a long "to do" list still clutched in our wrinkly, liver-spotted hands.

Think about your retired friends, and you will probably find both types. I certainly do. But I will only mention a few of the non-quiet, non-desperate ones because there's little to learn from the others. Eddie is an example. A retired Chief U. S. Probation Officer in Baton Rouge, Louisiana, he started a lawn care business when he retired and now he and his employees spend a lot of time making money on mowers. But Eddie also found there are a lot of elderly folks in his area, often widows, who simply can't afford lawn care, at least not to the degree that makes them feel proud of their lawn's appearance. So, Eddie began doing part of his work pro bono, as we say in the legal business. For tax and liability purposes, it was safer for him to formalize those arrangements, and Joshua's Ministry of Mowing was born.

Or retired teacher and coach Wayne Bennett in my native area of southern West Virginia. He genuinely likes meeting people and talking with them about our hometown, so, investing a small amount of money in a microphone, he began a podcast interviewing locals. When he had me in, we sat at his dining room table for about an hour and just chatted. It was that simple, and we both enjoyed it. Thousands of people listen to each episode because they almost always hear a familiar name. Or Goffinet McLaren, former Aer Lingus flight attendant originally from Carrickfergus, Ireland, who retired to Litchfield Beach, South Carolina and began a local beach cleanup group and campaign against plastic pollution. Or David Perdue, a retired web developer who used his skills to bring us the definitive Charles Dickens information page, suitably called *The Charles Dickens Page*. Or David Powell, a writer originally from Salem, West Virginia who almost singlehandedly brought the sport of Irish Road Bowling (Google it!) to the United States in areas that aren't pockets of Irish ex-pats.

What do these folks have in common? I happen to know them all personally. But more than that, in retirement they all have something about which they are *passionate*. They do what they do not for money, but for the love of the thing. All these examples help others in some way and helping others is important. Even if your passion is something that is for you and you alone, pursue it. Golf (just don't expect me to join you). Crochet. Make wreaths or birdhouses. Garden. Travel. Metal detect (count me in!). People make fun of some of these hobbies but that's none of their business. Volunteer. There is some organization out there that needs your help, and you don't have to be in charge. Okay, you were a high-powered executive or fashion designer or nursing supervisor most of your career, but there is a sense of serenity and pleasure in being asked to help set up tables and chairs and serve spaghetti at a shelter once a week without having to make additional decisions.

Of course, that doesn't preclude continuing to make money from your passion. If it can be done for profit in a way that doesn't suck all the joy out of it for you, forge ahead! So many things can even be done from home now, such as tutoring students around the world. Take a painting or pottery or fly-fishing class at the local community college. Or teach one! Sometimes retailers even offer classes free to spark interest. Now is your chance to indulge your "I don't know if I would like so-and-so, but I always wanted to try it" to find out. If it turns out to not be your thing, then don't be afraid to drop it and try something new. These days, the choices are endless and don't have to break the bank.

Maybe you would like to write. For a lot of people, the very suggestion seems daunting. Go into it with the idea that *this is just for myself,* and I have no expectations of seeing my work published. That takes the pressure off. Write about what you like, or what you know, or what you would LIKE to KNOW. There is more on this in the next chapter, when I introduce *The Book of the Still Living.*

Writing is my passion. If you haven't found yours, you have work to do. "My passion is spending time with my family by running errands and playing chauffeur and providing free babysitting services for my adult kids and grandkids and even great grandkids" is all well and good, but make sure it isn't just a cop out. Is your health important? Is your financial stability important? Are your family relationships important? Of course, they are. But without being seasoned with passion, even those are less satisfying. The day you no longer have something you are passionate about to look forward to is the day you stop looking forward at all.

3. PUSH YOURSELF

If life were meant to be easy, it wouldn't be so hard. If it were meant to be safe, it wouldn't be so dangerous. Squeeze what is hard and dangerous out of life, and all you have left are lemon rinds. They say those are good for deodorizing your garbage disposal, but I can't think of much else.

Stop pushing yourself to exercise and you get flabby and unhealthy. That applies to everything you've got, physically, mentally, spiritually, emotionally, socially, and any other -ly word you want to add. Sexually, even. Use it or lose it isn't just a catchy phrase. Without being pushed, your muscles, mind, spirit, relationships, and *even your genitals* will atrophy. Pushing yourself is not comfortable, nor is it meant to be. *But wait! Isn't comfort what we worked all those years to obtain, now that we're old?* you ask? Not at the expense of the time you have left. There will be plenty of time for comfort without negative consequence when you're dead, if one believes in an afterlife (which I do, for the record).

If you can walk a quarter mile, you can likely work up to a half mile. If you do ten curls at 20 pounds, you can likely work up to 20 curls at 30 pounds. It doesn't have to be done all at once, or even over a week or month, but when whatever you are doing becomes so easy that it doesn't cause you to "feel" it, that's a sign to move on and step up.

If you can see a screen and push keys, you can learn to use a computer, even if you are 90 and have never used so much as a Univac with punch cards before. The Dutch Longitudinal Internet Study for the Social Sciences found that respondents over 65 who showed more frequent internet use, specifically searching for information and using email, consuming media, and using social applications, reported higher levels of cognitive engagement, being open to new experiences. "It's not just watching a screen that is psychologically important, it's what kind of screen," said Ted Schwaba, a researcher at the University of Texas Austin who was a lead author in the project. You need things that are stimulating and engaging, things that make you think and become more curious.

Never traveled alone? Begin with an overnight bus tour. They are abundant and inexpensive. Get help from a travel club, such as the AAA or something similar. If you have been half of a couple for most of your life, it is difficult to begin to do things alone. "I hate to go out to eat or to a movie by myself" is a common and understandable complaint among the recently widowed or divorced. I know. I have been there. You must decide: I will either push myself, or I, mind, muscle and genitals, will atrophy.

Let's see...we've covered the gym, the internet, and going out to eat, so what's left. Oh...people. This is the tough one for me, being a natural introvert.

I may be overly optimistic, but I assume at least a few people I know in real life will read this book, and say, "Introvert? Yeah, right!" Those are the ones who know me from professional, civic, or other areas of my life where it is my job to be social. I can be an organizer, storyteller, "startup guy" as one friend used to say. I can walk into a room and present one of my programs for a hundred people without a second thought (and regularly do just that) and then schmooze and chat up every one of them during the coffee break. It's my job, and after years of practice I have (ahem) become good at it. But if, for example, my wife suggests we have dinner with a couple I haven't already known since Apolo Ohno last won gold in the Winter Olympics, I get anxious.

For some of you social butterfly types, this part isn't a problem. My stepson (the term usually followed by "the lawyer" when he comes up in conversation, especially when I am threatening a company that has done...me...wrong about something), while in college, visited our beach townhome for just a few days and knew more people here in that time than I do after 14 years. Both my brothers-in-law seem to think the natural thing to do when encountering another human is to strike up a conversation. And it is natural, *for them*. Doing anything different would be uncomfortable, unnatural. Since retiring and no longer having to interact with people every day, it is all too easy to convince myself I now deserve the comfort of not engaging with people. It shows, and it's bad for me. Look, I didn't say I follow all these rules, alright? But I know I must push myself. Through death and being dropped for less inevitable reasons, my friend bench could become very shallow ideed. I must push myself.

4.   STOP BEING A SCOREKEEPER

ALL THINGS I HAVE HEARD: *Darn it. She insisted on paying for my coffee, so next time I will have to pay for hers. But what if she also orders a scone as well? When we sold Mom's house, my siblings didn't reimburse me for last year's taxes on it, that I paid out of my own pocket. We like the McVanwinkles and always had a good time but stopped inviting them over because they seldom reciprocated. Wait a minute…we watched YOUR show four nights last week, and mine only three. That one friend always seems to be finished for the evening and has to leave just before it's his round for pints, now doesn't he? Why doesn't she ever buy the first tank of gas, because that's sometimes all it takes for the trip? I treated those guys well when we went to New York for three nights and THOUGHT we had agreed that someone else would pay next time, and I don't mean a $100 daytrip to Niagara Falls.*

She said something, and the more I thought about it, I wondered if it was a slight of some kind. Then it happened again just two years later. That did it. I didn't ask questions to clarify, I just ended our contact. If she wants me, she knows where to find me.

Mom always liked him better, I know, but shouldn't things have been divided equally?

The scorekeeping never ends. None of us would need Ginkgo Biloba supplements to improve our memory if scientists could only synthesize low dose resentment extract, because that stuff never gets forgotten. It's a lifelong game, and not divided into innings. The numbers on the scorecard just keep adding up. It's human nature.

Our ancient selves had to be competitive for food and other elements of basic survival. Each relationship had to be continually evaluated on that basis. Neanderthals Og and Ogla probably didn't sit down and discuss how to turn one three-toed sloth into a "win/win" situation. She clubbed him and took it, so she won. Today, most of our partners of whatever degree aren't threatening us with abandonment to the elements and death, but the primal instinct remains.

We are competitors by nature. We want to win. We don't want to feel someone has taken advantage of us. It's a fine line to tread, because it is all based on perception that others do things consciously to beat us. In other words, it's just that: about *us*. No matter if it's paying for lunch or buying a pint or the price tag of presents bought for one another's grandkids' confirmations, we remember and compare instead of appreciating things in their moments.

The wise adage "forgive and forget" isn't part of human nature. That scorecard is always clutched in our hot little hand. The key is what we do with it. My prescription, which I assure you I follow at least 43% of the time:

1. Call yourself out on it. After reading this, keep the word *scorekeeping* in your mind, and learn to recognize it in your thinking. You may find yourself doing it more than you think.
2. Weigh the costs and benefits. Okay, I know I end up paying for two pints to his one, and that I offer to buy lunch, but he seldom does. Do you enjoy one another's company, though? If so, consider it an investment, however reluctant.
3. Never mark the score until you have communicated about it. No one can or should be expected to read our minds. If we always offer to pay, and someone always accepts, who's fault (if there is one) is that? "Hey, I think I paid last time. You're not leavin' just before you buy a round, are ye, lad? (It's hard for me to think of that one in anything but an Irish accent, having spent as much time in Irish pubs as I have in my life) So, we agreed the next trip is yours. Where and

when, and do you want help planning it? How do we want to divvy up buying the gasoline? Get specific agreements. Otherwise, the score you assign isn't valid. That goes two ways. Own up to your own transgressions and apologize for them.

4. Give everyone a chance for redemption. You have probably said or done things that others marked on their little scorecards without meaning to do so or even being aware of it. If it's something that still bothers you and impacts your relationships, needs to be addressed and resolved if possible.

When my daughter was born, I made my lifelong best friend her Godfather. But, around that time, our lives took different directions and we mostly fell out of contact, not through any conflict, but just went our separate ways. He never sent her a single Christmas or birthday card. She didn't even hear from him when her mother died. My daughter is now approaching 40, but I still resent that. I should have a conversation with him. Dude, that's your goddaughter, regardless of how sparse our contact is now. Maybe he doesn't have the same concept of what that role means? Or does he just not care? I guess I'll never know unless I have the discussion, but it's hard to approach someone like that after all these years. Still, I would like to have some explanation. Some peace on it. I don't want to shame him. I just want to understand. I've tried to let it go, but it's still there. -Male

5. Try to avoid *You never* and *You always,* both in thought and speech, because they are seldom valid. Few things are so absolute.
6. When all else fails, you may have to resort to that old Appalachian explanation and apology for all bad behavior: *That's just the way he or she is.* So fatalistic. Some folks aren't going to change. It could be a psychological issue that goes much deeper than the check at the Dubliner, something far beyond our understanding, much less control. If the outcome is not worth the resentment, then maybe it is, indeed, time to say the relationship is not worth the

investment. Remember this step begins with when all else fails.

That's all a hard ask since we are so evolutionarily hardwired to compete, and to keep those scores. These steps won't always work, but you won't know without trying them. I know my comfort level with people who aren't scorekeepers is considerably greater than with others who embrace it.

The advent of social media has allowed us to continue scorekeeping that should have ended before the dawn of disco. We can now scroll through the "best lives" of classmates with whom we competed and never settled old scores all those years ago. Take those people who looked down on this geeky, nearsighted, bookish, nonathletic coal miner's son from up the holler back in the mid-1970s and with whom I have not personally interacted in all those intervening years: I am supposed to EMBRACE them at our upcoming fiftieth reunion? After seeing all their photos of boat outings and European trips and backyard barbeques on $30,000 patios?

You haven't done so bad yourself. I bet a couple of them are jealous of some of the things you have done in life. That scorecard? Let it go, y'all.

5. FOCUS ON RELATIONSHIPS AND EXPERIENCES, NOT STUFF

It sometimes seems our lives are spent in constant pursuit of stuff, right up until the end. But then, we leave this world as bigger, hairier, and less attractive versions of the same way we entered it, with exactly the same amount of stuff, if you don't count artificial hips and pacemakers.

You probably know people, especially seniors, who make life decisions based on preservation of their *stuff* instead of quality of life. Accumulated detritus fills every garage, attic, basement, and backyard shed in the world. We just can't seem to help ourselves. When Sandy and I married, I lived in a 3,000+ square foot house (plus 800 square foot workshop) in which my late wife and I had raised our two daughters. Every square inch was filled with that life.

Tons of Toys. Copiousness of Clothing. Billions of Books. Cascades of Cookware. Plethoras of Posters. Even worse, I am a natural "collector," and so was my late wife. My wife Sandy, on the other hand, lived in a house that was uncluttered, peaceful, serene. Our task was to sell both those houses in West Virginia and combine our lives in our newly built 1,600 square foot 3-story townhome at the beach for which we were buying all new furniture. I cannot think of an exercise more daunting, heart-rending, freeing, and cathartic all at once than that. Truckloads of things went to the landfill and to the charity shops. I hosted a "take what you want" evening for selected friends and relatives. The rest, including a Dodge pickup truck, was auctioned for a *total* of around $4,000. A moving auction seems like a good solution, and it can be, if you assume you will walk away with a fraction of what the auction company pockets.

But I was free to move on. My new garage cabinets are full of tools that I may sometime still need, and the attic is still stacked with plastic totes, but fewer than before, because I am in what I call my Phase of De-acquisition. Every time my kids and/or grandkids visit, something from the attic goes back with them. They can choose it, or I do. As the grandkids get older, I can determine their interests and act accordingly. One gets my coin collection. Another gets my political campaign buttons. Yet another gets my…somethings. (She's only five, so we'll see where her interests may lead.)

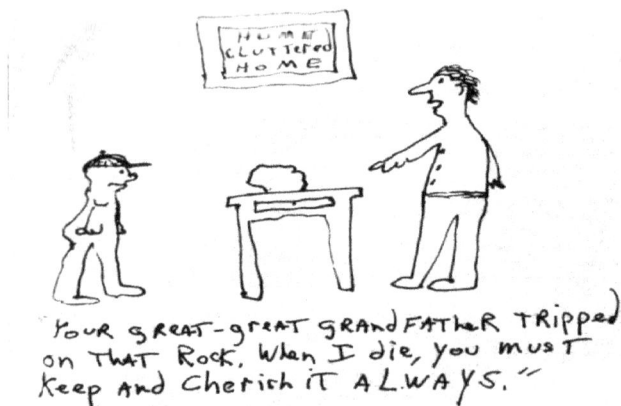

YouR gReAT-greAT gRANd FATHeR TRIpped on ThaT Rock, When I die, you musT keep And Cherish iT ALWAYS."

I hate being alone since my husband died. The house is too much for me to handle, and in the winter sometimes I don't see anyone for days on end. My son wanted me to sell the house and move into a small townhome near him where it's much warmer and he would be nearby, but what would I do will all my furniture? I have had some of it for more than 60 years! -Female

Making life decisions based on 1950s Montgomery Ward bedroom suites makes perfect sense, right?

Sell stuff you don't use and have a good time with the proceeds. Make it your determined mission to find friends or family who actually want old items that may have sentimental value. Keep the things that have real meaning to you and are seen and used instead of buried in the closet. You will be disappointed to find how little some of those things you paid such good money for during the Carter administration are worth, and that no one wants them. But…but…do you have any idea how much I spent on those Beanie Babies? Those Precious Moments and Hummel figurines? The cigarette smoke I inhaled playing Longaberger Bingo to win those baskets? My Norman Rockwell collector plates? That pitchfork belonged to MY GRANDFATHER, for heaven's sake. Anything that old *must* be valuable!

I am not your appraiser, and it is possible that some select items on that list may be worth something to someone. Find out who and try to put them together. Want to embrace legacy? Label things you decide to keep so your descendants will know why they were kept, and why they are important to you. That will help make their decisions easier and pass knowledge down to the next generation about what may be worthwhile, but ultimately it will be up to them. Go to an antique store and you will find baskets of beautiful 100-year-old-plus sepia photographs of handsome families in their Sunday best for a couple bucks each. Those people likely have living descendants who have never seen the images and who would be thrilled to do so, but for the want of writing names, dates, and location on the back it won't happen. That is so sad to me that I occasionally adopt one and make copies for my relatives as, saying it is of our long-lost ancestors. I mean, it *could* be, right?

No one can prove me wrong, and everybody's happy.

Charity shops and sales may be your last chance. If no takers, as painful as it is, reconcile yourself to the fact that tons of cherished Greatest Generation and Baby Boomer possessions go to landfills every day. I agree that it's sad but see for yourself. Go to a few estate sales and see what sells (and for what price) and what doesn't. You will be convinced. Just don't bring someone else's stuff back home with you! The same will happen with your things. Do yourself and your loved ones a favor. Don't leave them to deal with the decisions and the uncertainty and guilt. Decide what's truly important to you and then sell-give-donate-trash, freeing yourself to live less encumbered. After you have foisted enough things off on your friends and family, only accumulate new things that you love, or you will have to start the process over. Then focus on experiences rather than stuff, giving and expecting to receive them as gifts. For your granddaughter's graduation, you could buy her a $5,000 used car, or take her to Paris for a week. Which will she tell her own grandchildren about someday when you're long gone? When asked what you want for your own 70th birthday, a bitchin' party down at the K of C hall with a polka band and kegs of Yuengling will make memories not only for you, but others.

Your kids will never have to guiltily send that party to the landfill because Goodwill won't take it, and that story about the Deacon getting caught eying one of the catering waitresses and his wife pouring salt on his slice of birthday cake could well outlive you.

6. DROP THE FAÇADE

Good grief, get over yourself. The time for posturing and one upmanship and caring about the appearance of importance and being better than everyone else should be long over for those of us staring into the abyss, don't you think? Everyone's job was important. The size of your 401k isn't anyone else's business, much less something to be broadcast. We're all in this old boat together now, and it's slowly sinking. How big your office was or your number of degrees or how many people you supervised won't serve as life preservers.

We seniors aren't impressed by much anymore, so is your boorish posturing worth it to only make yourself feel better?

That sounds mean, I know. Look around at an assemblage of seniors, though, and you will often find a cacophony of self-importance, so much *what I did* and *what I have* that it would be more pleasant to stay home. Do yourself a real favor and relish the fact that facades are no longer necessary. You don't need to pretend to like chardonnay or being on the Community Concert Series board or every little kid you encounter in public or reading significant books or even your own nephew. No, you are not the Great Oracle and Font of All Knowledge Who Is Always Right Because You Have Done and Read So Much, so don't pretend to be. In fact, you shouldn't pretend at all. It's freeing. Try it. (But read Rule # 7 and don't use Rule #6 as an excuse to be a jerk, okay? There's a difference.)

While we all hope our romantic relationships last a lifetime, there are many instances in which people are profoundly unhappy, enduring emotional and even physical abuse for years, but can't bring themselves to drop the Cleaver image of the happy family to escape it. While all those years of familial, social, and financial intertwining may seem impossible to untangle, seek support and find the courage to put your own well-being over the perceptions you have so painfully maintained while you still have some time left to enjoy. We have already referenced Bronnie Ware's excellent book *The Top Five Regrets of the Dying: A Life Transformed by the Dearly Departing* (Hay House, August 2019). The number one regret?

"I wish I'd had the courage to live a life true to myself, not the life others expected of me."

There's no more to say, unless you want to know Bronnie Ware's full list: 1. I wish I'd had the courage to live a life true to myself, not the life others expected of me. 2. I wish I hadn't worked so hard. 3. I wish I'd had the courage to express my feelings. 4. I wish I'd stayed in touch with my friends. 5. I wish I'd let myself be happier.

NOW there's no more to say about it.

7. AND YOUR SENSE OF PRIVILEGE

An open letter to participants in the multiple golf cart and pleasure boat political candidate parades and flotillas in 2020:

I don't care about your politics. I really don't. Make your own decision based on your beliefs about who can do the best job for our country and promote it. Be proud of it. But those overtly tribal 'look at us, we've made it, and we don't care about anyone else and ---- your feelings' displays tinged with intolerance are bad for all of us senior citizens. Sincerely, Danny

Do we really want to reinforce the stereotype of 'old, racist, homophobic Baby Boomers' among the succeeding generations who will shortly be in control of everything, including decisions sure to impact important aspects of senior care and standards of living? Treating younger people and their views with derision does not seem to be a winning strategy for those who are on the verge of having mobility and continence issues, if you ask me.

At least the golf carts, unlike some of the boats, didn't sink, unless maybe one went into the fountain at The Villages.

Old people complaining about younger people isn't new. I am, in addition to being a writer and nongolfer, a corporate trainer (see www.favoritetrainers.com) and have taught a class on generational communication for years, using this quote, attributed (probably incorrectly) to Socrates (469-399 B.C.): "The children now love luxury; they have bad manners, contempt for authority; they show disrespect for elders and love chatter in place of exercise. Children are now tyrants, not the servants of their households. They no longer rise when elders enter the room. They contradict their parents, chatter before company, gobble up dainties at the table, cross their legs, and tyrannize their teachers." In the class, I first show the quote and ask participants about whom it was most likely said. Invariably, each generation believes it was said about the ones following them instead of by someone who lived almost twenty-five hundred years ago. I suspect it's always been such, with my great-grandfather complaining about my grandfather being interested in motor cars instead of safer and more dependable horses, and my great-grandmother scandalized that my grandmother wore shoes that laced instead of buttoned.

As a little thought exercise, let's turn this around just a bit: "The senior citizens now love luxury; they have bad manners, contempt for authority; they show disrespect for younger people and love chatter in place of exercise. Seniors are now tyrants, not the servants of their households. They contradict everyone, chatter before company, gobble up dainties at the table, cross their legs, and tyrannize their families."

From a non-senior citizen's viewpoint, it might be hard to contradict that statement. I live in a community with lots of retirees, and I see it every day. When I overhear senior citizens complain about younger people having a sense of "privilege and entitlement," I just about spew out my coffee (if I am at Barnes and Nobel) or beer (if I am almost anywhere else I frequent). These are the same jerks complaining that the fire lane in front of Food Lion is already completely full of golf carts and there isn't any room left for theirs. The people who let their doggies do what doggies doo on the sidewalk without remediation, while posting "No trespassing. Owner is armed" signs on their own lawns. The people who deserve their healthcare and Social Security while voting for those who would deny those things to others. The people who cheer at footage of a Border Patrol agent lassoing someone trying to cross, while hiring a young mother to clean their house at a fraction of what the service is worth because the woman is undocumented.

At almost every meeting I attend of whatever organization dominated by older males, the one-upmanship reminds me of a pen full of Banty roosters. (Remember I grew up on a farm) Then, they wonder why they lack younger members. "These young people today just aren't civic minded!" Dang, dudes. I can hardly stand to be around you myself, and I have far less to do at home than those youngsters.

A sense of privilege and entitlement, indeed. Privilege to disregard parking and intersection rules, drive golf carts where they are prohibited, save 18 lounge chairs on the Lido Deck for your whole family even though some of them won't show up for hours, cut line at the theater, loudly voice your opinions on politics, people's dress, the price of a cheeseburger, slow service, sports, and everything else under the sun in public places, not lift both lids in a public bathroom, dressing too casually for the location, not attending to personal hygiene (body odor), having the back of one's vehicle covered in stickers specifically meant to offend someone, refusing to use hearing aids if needed, holding everyone up because you didn't even begin looking for your money/credit card/ID/discount card until you were asked for them at the front of the line, dominating conversations with how important you once were in your job or how successful your current investing may be, making racist or homophobic remarks at the Thanksgiving table, not carrying your fair share at work if you are still employed…need I go on?

Expecting to be respected and catered to simply because of one's age is the very privilege and entitlement for which I hear Millennials and Gen Z so often belittled.

Your beliefs and opinions are valid, *for you*. Look around. In general, Millennials and Gen Z are less prejudiced, bigoted, racist, and homophobic than Boomers and Gen X. You aren't going to reverse that. For example, according to the Pew Research Center, Americans opposed legal same-sex marriage by a margin of 60% to 31% in 2004. A June 2023 poll found a whopping 71% of Americans support it. And, even more significant, here are the results of the First Official "How Much of What Other Consenting Adults Do in Their Bedrooms is None of Your Business Poll:" an incredible 100%! (Okay, there wasn't really a poll. I didn't need one, and you don't either.)

Just because half the people with whom you attended prom are no longer with us doesn't make you King or Queen of it, and even senior citizen Jorge Mario Bergoglio said, "Who am I to judge?" Intolerance can become obsession can become hate, and it eats people alive, robbing them and those around them of joy. You have a choice in the way you interact with the world. You can assume the privilege and entitlement of old age and reinforce negative stereotypes of seniors, or you can decide that you are not too old to learn a new skill.

That skill is called empathy. And your lack of it negatively affects you own life, those of your younger loved ones, and the relationships between you. Is it worth it? Even if you decide the answer is yes, your behavior still hurts the rest of us by feeding the stereotype.

Please stop it.

8. LIVE IN THE REAL WORLD, NOT THE SCREEN WORLD OR THE PAST WORLD

The Screen World: The Pew Research Center is one of the most well-respected social issue and demographic research "think tanks" in the world. Its analysis of the U. S. Census Bureau/Bureau of Labor Statistics American Time Use Survey found that, from 2005 to 2015, older Americans increased their daily screen time by a full 27%, and there is no reason to suspect it hasn't continued to increase since then. During the same period, reading time decreased 13%, socializing 9%, and other leisure 6%. Today's 18-year-old will stare at a screen for *28 years* by the time she or he is 80.

Brethren and, um, Sistern, Ah am guilty! Not so much with television (ours is seldom turned on until 6:00 pm for the news, but then it is usually on until bedtime, which is still too much), but I can't seem to put down that wretched phone and checking Faccbook, Messenger, Instagram, LinkedIn, and my email.

First, television: ours is the TV generation, right? Anyone else have a behemoth dark wood black-and-white Zenith that picked up three stations, and one of those required running out in the snow to turn the antenna? Things have changed, and for our mental health not necessarily for the better. A 2022 study on the connection between screen time and cognition (39) borders on frightening. Surveying almost 150,000 test subjects in the United Kingdom 60+ in age found that the amount of time passively watching television is associated with increased risk of dementia, while using a computer in cognitively stimulating activity did not. Both, though, are associated with all the physical health risks of sitting: Diabetes, heart disease, stroke, loss of muscle tone, and all the other "sitting is the new smoking" maladies. They're real.

It's not just brain and body rotting. It can also harm your mental health, largely depending on what you watch. A steady viewing diet of scary, negative content without resolution and a high degree of uncertainty about outcome, a.k.a. *the news*, can lead to anxiety and even depression, as well as obsessive thinking. Compared to the days of Walter Cronkite, there are innumerable news outlets today that must compete for viewership, and many do that by trying to out-outrage one another. No wonder we come away with fear and loathing. Incongruently, perhaps, I recommend watching something: *The Brainwashing of My Dad* (2015) is a documentary by Jen Senko describing her father Frank's descent into fear and anxiety from watching too much cable news, and his ultimate redemption. It is narrated by Matthew Modine and has an appearance by the iconic professor Noam Chomsky.

I have seen it happen. It changes people. Though I haven't found similar studies on watching grisly true crime show after true crime show, I doubt that's good for you, either. My own personal research indicates a profound difference in mood after watching a couple episodes of *Keeping Up Appearances* vs. one of *Monster: The Jeffrey Dahmer Story*. Big surprise.

How much television is okay? Probably less than you (and I) watch now. *The English Longitudinal Study of Aging*, referenced several times already, found in 2008-09 and again in 2014-15 that those who watched 3.5 hours or more of television per day had an average decline of 8-10% in word and language-related memory. Don't watch more than three hours of television a day and make most of it pleasant.

Now, the phone: Device addiction is associated with depression and anxiety and disproportionately victimizes lonely people, making seniors particularly vulnerable. According to research from Reviews.org quoted in an article by L'Oréal Thompson Payton in *Fortune Magazine* (July 19, 2023), Americans interact with their phones 144 times a day for a total of 4 hours and 25 minutes.

What's the payoff for that much of our lives? You must answer that yourself. But it isn't just "habit" or boredom. It sets up the dynamic of true addiction, rewarding your brain with a tiny hit of dopamine each time you unlock and scroll. Instead of satisfying, it generates a desire to continue. How to break this addiction? It may help to first find out just how bad it is, and most phones have a mechanism to log their use. *Be prepared for shock.*

Then, divide that amount in half. Ration it out throughout your day however best fits your schedule. Work toward a goal of giving yourself 30 minutes in the morning, 30 in the evening, and a quick check midday. Turn off your notifications so you control the device instead of the other way around. And don't feel panicked if you fail to have your phone on your person or within reach every minute. We made it through the first half of our lives without it always in our hot little hands just fine, remember? Keep it somewhere in the house where you must make at least some effort to access it. At any time, of course, if you really need to know the hours of Minelli's Restaurant and Pizza Carryout, located at 3858 Sullivant Avenue in Columbus, Ohio, go ahead and search it, but then put your phone back down to process the devastating news that it is permanently closed, according to my phone just now.

Social media is both a blessing and a curse. We are in touch with far more of our family and friends because we have this relatively new technology, and that can be grand. I still communicate with some of my high school friends and former students solely because they are on social media; we would never have remained attached otherwise. Many have reconnected with me, seen something (usually political) they disliked, and now we are severed forevermore. My personal social media rules: If I see you post something with which I disagree, I will scroll by and not react. If it's so outrageous that it indicates the person and I are not compatible in beliefs (such as being racist or homophobic, for example), I quietly block the connection without reaction or announcement. When it comes to my posted opinions, I expect the same courtesy.

Now The Past World: It's no secret that, when seniors get together, they talk about the past. There's just so much more of it than the future for us, right? But if you dwell there too much, you are living your leftovers instead of dining on the present. Nostalgia is comforting and may help shield us from the anxiety of present-day challenges. Much of it can also be your subconscious attempt to rewrite the past to deal with pain and disappointment. I use two sayings often: 1. Nostalgia is like a grammar lesson. You find the present tense and the past perfect, and 2. (as the old barber said) It's okay to look backward. Just don't stare.

There is wisdom in both. Through years of that subconscious rewriting, the past can become so warm and comfortable and safe. Our family all got along, we were poor but happy, we did almost everything together, people were kinder to one another, an 18¢ hamburger at the Burger Boy Food-O-Rama was an utterly delicious treat, and the music was so much better.

Much of that is the result of subconscious revision, except, of course, the music being better part. How many times one can watch reruns of the *Andy Griffith Show* and still get anything out of them? (Answer for my brother: infinity. Answer for me: zero.) Most likely, your life today is filled with more opportunities, more comfort, more information, more financial resources, and more culture than ever before. There have been wonderful movies, television shows, cars, and everything else made since the end of the disco era. Explore them. Reject what you don't like but keep an open mind. Be aware of how much you slip into longing for the past, how much "retro" you surround yourself with every day, how much of your conversation is taken up with what is done and won't be changed instead of what you can still plan in the future.

Now excuse me while I watch my daily *Jonny Quest* rerun on YouTube. Best theme music ever!

THE TAKEAWAY

I know it's a shock to find this out after all these years, but you're never going to have the perfect spouse, children, siblings, grandchildren, in-laws, body, vacation, house, financial ledger, golf game, sex life, retirement package, faith community, civic organization, hobby, schedule, group of friends, or anything else. Even your dog with whom you share the closest thing to unconditional love in your life will eventually get old and develop bladder stones and pee on the sofa and require a $6,000 surgery more than once and eventually die in your arms (My wife and I know. I almost cried writing that). But every single one of those things (and others) bring you joy, at least occasionally. Determine who you really are and what is truly important to you and embrace them all today, despite their imperfections and challenges. Failing to do so will leave you joyless and filled with regret on your deathbed. Threading the needle between dropping the façade and being your true self while not being a privileged jerk to other people is possibly our last great mission in life. "I ain't' living my life for others" is healthy. "I live in such a way that others won't have anything to do with me" is not. "Now that I'm old, I can say and do what I want" is valid, but it always is, at any age. It was always your choice.

Most of your legacy has already been built. If the façade-less "true you" is a bitter, angry scorekeeper, there is still time to change. "Ha! I bullied people and cut off my friends because they did things I didn't like, and will try to set it up so that I still do that from the grave!" You can try, but remember the only thing you are likely to leave that can't end up on the discount table at an estate sale is the memory others have of you. That's about all we really can influence right down to the very end, which brings us, literally, to the final chapter.

I am told I came into the world naked, bald, chubby, penniless, and complaining. Look's like I'm going out that way, too. -Male

8 THE END

You're going to die, and it will probably be sooner than it has been. But there are things you can do to make the time you have left better.

One of those things is to do all you can to make your wishes for how you die known, but with the understanding that, no matter what you do, things may not necessarily go as planned. We have all seen many more movie deaths than actual deaths, and the two often have little in common.

What is it like to die? There are as many answers as there are people. Step in front of a speeding bus and you may not even notice it. Suffer through chemo and radiation for months to find they were unsuccessful or lose muscle control due to ALS and the process is ever present. It's strange that most of us understand so little about death, this fellow traveler who has been with us, either as a stalker or companion depending on how you look at it, since the day we were born. We can't even agree on what constitutes dying. Not so very long ago, if a person stopped breathing and had no pulse, that was that. Today, with ventilators and defibrillators, it may be more complicated, and even ambiguous. While those interventions often don't work, there are thousands of people walking around today who could be considered certified members of the Lazarus Club.

There is so much grey area that doctors at Harvard Medical School felt a uniform definition of death was needed, and in 1968 developed criteria that included the loss of brain stem reflexes. The Uniform Determination of Death Act is a model law that has been adopted by most states and specifies EITHER 1) irreversible cessation of circulatory and respirator functions, OR 2) irreversible cessation of all functions of the entire brain, including the brain stem. That sounds straightforward (even with the big EITHER/OR), but how is the term *irreversible* determined in a hospital room crammed with every possible machine to take over bodily functions but no crystal ball?

There is discussion of changing *irreversible* to *permanent*, implying that breathing and pulse will not restart on their own, and won't be artificially restarted because doing so will not restore a meaningful quality of life. That, in many circumstances, is a call determined by available resources (you have a heart attack while spelunking a mile underground), or by your advance directives. Absent those, it could also be made by your crystal ball-less next-of-kin or healthcare professionals. Is it possible that factors like expense, making organs available for transplant, tiredness, lateness of the hour, type of health insurance, the patient's socioeconomic status, level of personal affinity or other factors may play a role in those decisions? Of course not. (-eyeroll-)

Even this standard is not uniform, and whether you are dead can vary depending on what state (of the Union) you happen to be in at the time. In New Jersey, for example, a person's family can prevent a declaration of death without "total brain death" criteria having been met, on religious grounds. If you are thinking that, given today's heart-and-lung-pumping technology this could have harrowing consequences fit for a Robin Cook thriller, you are correct.

Absent a sudden extensive injury, the dying body's systems may slow down gradually. Your pulse and blood pressure decrease and weaken; blood moves around lazily, and your brain receives less oxygen, affecting thoughts and reactions. You are tired and may sleep a lot (which may be increased by pain medications). Your appetite decreases as your digestive processes slow and you produce less waste. Your skin may become pallid and thinner and then blotchy as cells stop regenerating. Breathing may become shallow, and alternately slow and quicken. Fluid gathers in your lungs, causing a rattling or gurgling sound. Your eyes may become glassy, your extremities cold to the touch, and you may become anxious and agitated, especially as you fight for breath. Some may become confused, even hallucinate (*or is it?* Most of us have heard stories of the dying apparently seeing and even talking with their deceased loved ones, giving rise to the notion that we see those we are about to join), or you may become calm and lose consciousness. Your senses and faculties fail, first hunger and thirst, then speech and vision. Hearing and touch can be the last to go, leaving open the question of how much someone otherwise unconscious can still sense another talking and feeling their hand being held. Eventually, your heart stops beating, you stop breathing, and within minutes your brain stops functioning due to lack of oxygen. Your mouth may fall open, your eyelids half close, and your sphincters may release whatever, if anything, they were holding back.

That's what happens to your body. But *what is it like to die?* What do you feel? Is it like drifting off to sleep? How much do we know about what is going on around us, even if we are no longer able to respond to it? If you are looking for concrete answers, I'm good, but not that good. Our ability to know is limited. If someone is unusually lucid up until the very end, she or he may describe their feelings, and some who have been resuscitated do as well.

The most common experiences mentioned include a feeling of leaving one's body (the most frequent) and even seeing that body lying in the hospital bed (and sometimes trying to return to it), ultra-heightened senses, seeing shining lights (or conversely traveling in a dark void), entering a tunnel, having a sense of peace, and communication with the dead, often loved ones but sometimes strangers. It also appears the likelihood and nature of such experiences may be related to one's spiritual beliefs before nearing the end. And the ever popular "my life flashed before my eyes?" While relatively rare, it has been reported, sometimes described as being like watching a movie. (My own personal experience with this is limited. Years ago, when building an addition onto my house, I tumbled headfirst onto a concrete slab eleven feet below when the sheet of subflooring I was nailing down flipped with me on it. I sustained some broken ribs and other injuries and was unconscious for a time. Instead of waking with a memory of sitting with Siskel and Ebert {both of whom now reside in the great beyond} eating popcorn and making snarky remarks about the movie of my life, the only thought I recalled about the moment of my falling was "Oh, shoot!" Or something close.)

The good news is that positive experiences seem to outnumber hellish ones about three-to-one, but that is subject to the limited information available, including a study republished by the National Library of Medicine's National Center for Biotechnology Information in 2023. (40)

Another scholarly review of published reports (41) reveals that, among more than a hundred cardiac arrest survivors participating in extensive interviews, almost half believed they had memories of their "time out," with seven main themes represented: fear, plants and/or animals, bright light, violence/persecution, a feeling of Deja-vu, family, and seeing or hearing actual events related to their resuscitation.

Some researchers believe there are biomedical explanations for all these reports, while others say some do not appear to be scientifically understandable with the information available. My own Celtic ancestors, not all that long ago, were very careful to give the spirit every opportunity to leave a loved-one's body, stowing the corpse near an open window or even stopping all the clocks and covering the mirrors in the house to keep said spirit from getting trapped in the house. Not…good…for…resale…value. I have been to a couple of wakes where the spirits flowed freely, but usually out in the funeral home or church parking lot.

For most of us, perceptions of what death is like have probably been influenced by the way it is portrayed on television and in movies, and deviation from those may disappoint us. Yes, I would really like for my family to wheel a big piece of Plexiglas in so I could put my palm on it with them taking turns doing the same on the other side while I say, "I have been, and always shall be your *husband, father, brother, cousin, friend, parishioner, customer at*

Tupelo Honey happy hour or whatever the case may be, but think about the logistics involved! Death is not even the only human activity that can disappoint us by the perception that "media portrayal equals reality." See Chapter 1, which was much more fun researching than this one.

With no expiration date digitally printed on some out-of-the-way and hard to read spot on our bodies, decisions about death may, ironically, be the most difficult of our lives. You would have to be Vulcan to be able to view it with complete logic and objectivity. Life is precious. It's the final thing we possess, and decisions about it may be irreversible. For people used to making rational choices after gathering all the facts (like me), we are frustrated when we hit such an impenetrable wall. You may well feel 100% confident that you know exactly what happens when you die. Good for you! I am sure that's comforting. There are many cases in which people live with that confidence their entire lives, but then, when death is imminent, still fear it.

Take, for example, the Puritan clergyman Increase Mather (1639 – 1723), president of Harvard from 1681 through 1701. He left lots of writing, so we have an abundance or original source material to learn about him. He was very much into persecuting Catholics (hey now, Increase, you're getting personal!) and anyone else not following his strict ideology and showed no mercy to those he felt committed sin, such as, oh, celebrating Christmas or drinking wine or doing anything but sitting in church on Sunday or women not having their bodies almost completely covered.

But what we remember old Increase most for today is his great disappointment over witch hunts declining in popularity in Europe, so much so that it was his mission to Make America Great Again by bringing back the practice on this side of the pond. His paper *Cases of Conscience Concerning Evil Spirits* tells how he convinced many of his followers that they had been downright negligent leaving so many witches unhunted, and they needed to do better. One of the trials he personally attended was that of fellow preacher George Burroughs, who had even filled in preaching for Mather in the pulpit a few times. Some of the locals who owed George money swore they saw him exhibit "extraordinary feats of strength" that could only be possible with assistance from Old Scratch himself. (Be careful how much y'all show off at the gym. You never know who's watching) George was found guilty of witchcraft and hanged on August 19, 1692. He recited the Lord's Prayer while standing on the ladder with the rope around his neck. The crowd began to wonder if a mistake hadn't been made, but our friend Increase's son Cotton, also a clergyman, was in the crowd and assured everyone *oh-don't-mind-that* and George swung...along with four others. They were buried so haphazardly that some parts protruded from the grave.

Why this history ramble? Because the last thing we know about old Increase is that, on his deathbed, this confident directed-by-Providence holier-than-all-y'all slave-owning pronouncer of justice was *scared to death to die.* According to contemporary accounts, he faced death with "desperate fear and trembling," tormented that he might be bound for Hell.

While some may believe they have had different experiences, no one I know and trust has ever died and come back with vivid memories of it so we can talk about the experience over a beer, allowing me to take notes on a bar napkin. Another reason the concept of death is so scary is that most of us live our lives trying to control all the various aspects of it, only in the end to be confronted by something over which we have none, and we don't much like it. So, no matter how firm your comfort with the concept of dying today while it is theoretical, prepare yourself for a possible change of attitude when it is more clearly approaching, and have some empathy for those doubts and that anxiety should they arise in your elder loved ones.

None of this fully answers the question, though, does it? We fear the unknown, and even though death is one of the most universal of humanity's shared experiences, it is still the undiscovered country, the great map-less journey, for each of us. Perhaps we will understand it all someday. Or maybe not. If you and I get to discuss it ("Dang. Can you believe we were so worried about *this*?") over a cold Smithwick's (with a lime slice) with all our other deceased loved ones sitting around us, I guess that would be heaven.

IT'S YOUR DECISION (SOMETIMES, MAYBE)

Is it, though? In a way, we feel we control some elements of our dying with our daily decisions over the years. Yes, you can eat a healthy diet, get plenty of exercise, never smoke or drink alcohol or use other drugs, avoid pollutants and UV rays, have regular checkups and everything else and still die young. There could be some small factory defect lurking in our DNA that could unexpectedly cause something to rupture or move or some cells to go crazy. Someone who is drunk or high or texting could run you down with his Toyota while you're biking. Many fatalistic folks believe that moment is preordained and nothing you do can change it. That's an easy position to defend, because how could you disprove it? No matter the manner of one's demise, someone can look and say, "It was her time."

The discussion can be muddied by the distinction of the term "natural death." To me, that's a misnomer. All death is natural, the most natural and inevitable thing about life. Even if one jumps off the edge of the Grand Canyon, the resulting injuries causing death will be *natural*. It has also been a common thing in human history for people under some circumstances to *choose* to stop living. But when life's "natural" end nears and a terminal diagnosis is given (either explicitly or implicitly), responses often take one of three forms:

1. Fight to delay it at all costs, no matter the amount of pain or disability. While the will to "fight" is personal, the decision to keep someone alive as long as medically possible may be made by someone else if the proper legal provisions are not in place. The first round of the fight is to force all the relevant information out of a system that often doesn't lend itself to being upfront with it. Doctors get no joy out of giving bad news, and some of them are horrible at communicating it (no offense, docs). You may not be able to think of all your questions at once, so write them down and continue the conversation with your doctor when you are ready. Remember that she cannot know and tell you exactly what the progression of your condition may be, or how long you have left under different scenarios. She will only be able to share her opinion given her own experience with patients, and every one of us is different. You may

hear things like "20% of people in this stage of your condition live for 6 months or less" or "There is a positive response to this treatment in about half the cases." That's not very satisfying, but it may truly be the best she can do.

I asked my doctor, Doc, how long do I have? Well, she said, I can't say for sure, but if I were you, I wouldn't buy any green bananas. -Male

This doesn't necessarily fit with our modern, rather arrogant idea of both life and death. We too often believe every obstacle can be overcome if only we have the resources and determination. Death ain't like that, friends. You can chase the latest drug or treatment or holistic lifestyle change or whatever. They may help. But someday, dudes and dudettes, as we have been repeating, you gonna die.

Common death-delaying treatments include chemotherapy and radiation, spending three to four hours three times a week connected to a dialysis machine, carrying an oxygen tank every step of the day, wearing a colostomy bag or urinary catheter, leg amputation, or heart or lung surgery, along with many others that significantly impact one's daily quality of life. None are painless, without risk, or guaranteed to work for any specified amount of time. A true "fighter" will also make all the changes necessary to prolong life, such as those involving diet, exercise, smoking, drinking, relationships, and medications. Why wait? Those are all battles we can wage today.

A determined attitude partnered with affirmative action to improve one's overall health is the first volley in the battle of prolonging your life. But remember the concept of "fight" connotes there being a winner and a loser. You will not ultimately "win" this fight. None of us will. Your fight, should you choose it, is to delay that bell going off as long as possible. Please don't be offended, but hearing someone say, "She lost her battle with cancer," for example, puts me on edge. She may, indeed, have fought valiantly and gone through hell to prolong her life. That's not losing. And never forget that no matter how many times you have told yourself and others you will "fight to the finish," you can always make different decisions as needed. They should always be yours to make if you are able, and your prearranged wishes should be followed if you are not.

There are potential pitfalls. A 2018 Scottish study by the UK's Macmillan Cancer Support organization showed that a "fighting attitude" could have a negative effect on terminal cancer patients' end of life experience. About 63% of the patients considered themselves "fighters," and were less likely than others to discuss and implement end-of-life plans, sometimes leading to unintended, undesired, and avoidable negative outcomes concerning pain management, hospice care arrangements, and other critical decisions. About a quarter of the "fighters" felt guilty about not being able to stay positive about their disease, and almost as many found it difficult to talk honestly about their feelings. (Study quoted in the *Independent*, May 15, 2018. Despite my German surname, the part of me that isn't Irish is mostly Scottish, and I just can't imagine Scottish men finding it difficult to talk about our feelings, can you? I will note that study was conducted the same year Irn-Bru changed its formula, so maybe there is a connection).

Bottom line: if you fight, know what you are fighting for, and, to the extent possible, what's ahead. To "win" isn't to "beat this thing." Every day is a win. You might have known courageous people who have simply become so exhausted with the fight that they only wanted it to end, and that's okay. *They didn't lose.*

2. Passively allow the process to take its course. With proper pain management and other interventions in place, this is a common choice for patients and their families. Balancing how much medical intervention and treatment to pursue in order to delay the inevitable may require adjusting to the situation. For example, you may need to decide between more complete pain relief or being able to be alert enough to communicate with your loved ones; whether to undergo painful surgery with no guarantee it will buy you more quality time, or where (hospital, home, or hospice) to spend your very last moments. And (repeat, repeat, repeat) these decisions are best made by *you* while you are still able to do so and revise as you wish.

You may have known someone who went through chemo and radiation treatments that possibly extended their life for a short time, but that time sucked. Deciding to forego those treatments to have shorter but potentially better time on the clock can be a very rational choice. The kicker is that there are also many people who endured that hell and eventually *did* get much better as a result, adding a significant amount of quality time to their lives. *Will it be worth it* is something you can't know for sure and can only weigh the evidence and odds in consultation with your doctor.

One of your options during the last stages of disease may be hospice care, either in-home or in a hospice facility (which could also be a nursing home), or a combination of the two. As your level of assistance needed increases, doing everything yourself or depending solely upon a loved one may not be desirable or even possible. While hospice care focuses on those nearing the end of life, that has an element of subjectivity.

To qualify, your doctor generally certifies that your life expectancy is six months or less, you accept palliative (or comfort) care instead of active and extensive treatment of your illness, and you sign a statement choosing hospice care instead of other Medicare-approved interventions for your related conditions. Medicare guidelines (as of this writing) are to provide two 90-day periods of hospice care followed by an unlimited number of 60-day benefit periods. A benefit period starts the day you begin hospice care and ends when your 90-day or 60-day benefit ends.

Palliative care, as defined by the NIH's National Institute on Aging, is "specialized medical care for people living with a serious illness, such as cancer or heart failure. Patients in palliative care may receive medical care for their symptoms (a)long with treatment intended to cure their serious illness. Palliative care is meant to enhance a person's current care by focusing on quality of life for them and their family." Compare that to the Medicare's requirement noted above that you "accept palliative (or comfort) care instead of care to cure your illness" to receive the hospice benefit, and you may find you need to consult your doctor about your diagnosis and how it relates to Medicare benefits.

The NIH clearly states that a person in palliative care *only* does not have to give up treatment that might cure a serious illness, but, if ongoing treatment for the primary illnesses is no longer working, the patient may transition into hospice care, which begins to focus more on comfort. This is one reason why the 6-months-or-less-left diagnosis is an important criterion.

When it comes to life, fear of the unknown, and family dynamics, the distinctions between these terms and criteria can complicate decisions. When a loved one is receiving hospice care at home and the family has been instructed about what happens as the patient is dying, it's still far too common for them to panic and do things like call for an ambulance to take the patient to the hospital ER. That is like allowing a full code to be called in the hospital on a loved one with no discernable brain activity, or not agreeing to remove the ventilator from someone in a similar state. Even patients who have requested hospice care sometimes change their minds and ask for every possible intervention in their last moments of lucidity.

No matter the finer points of the definition, hospice care is meant for those no longer being aggressively treated to cure a disease, either because treatments are no longer working, or, like Art Buchwald, the patient has chosen not to pursue them. Art, (1925-2007) was one of my favorite writers and humorists. He became diabetic and, as a result, had a leg amputated and required kidney dialysis. By the time he was interviewed by Diane Rehm in February 2006, he had decided to stop dialysis and live his best life (which, for Art, meant leaving hospice care and spending time at McDonald's, among other things) for whatever time he had left, which turned out to be about 11 months.

What are the ethical considerations of choosing to discontinue treatment, either for yourself or being required to make that decision for a loved one? Some people irrationally consider refusing to pursue every possible treatment to be a form of suicide. Everyone is entitled to her or his personal beliefs, of course, but the late theologian Robert C. Sproul, founder of Ligonier Ministries, put it this way. "I don't want to have this sense that I'm obligated to go through all of these extraordinary means to preserve my life," he wrote. In my own particular faith, the Catechism of the Catholic Church says, "Discontinuing medical procedures that are burdensome, dangerous, extraordinary, or disproportionate to the expected outcome can be legitimate; it is the refusal of 'overzealous' treatment." It's not a sin to die. Many very, very devout people have done it over the years, and more do every day.

3. Take active measures to end one's life. At this point, some readers may take a judgmental and black/white attitude without nuance, but dying is as individual a thing as living, and one-size-fits-all pronouncements fail. Our technology has advanced to the point that death gets harder to define. Most (but not all) people would agree that withdrawing care (ventilator, etc.) from someone who has lain with no identifiable brain activity for days and whose organs are shutting down one by one is not murder. A few generations ago, those folks may have already been buried and their spouses remarried in the amount of time high-tech intervention is often employed today, so the argument could be made that *keeping them alive with no hope of improving is the unnatural act.* Have your advance directives in place!

While you are still able to make your own decisions, right up to the end, can there be instances when a rational person can choose the time of his or her death instead of awaiting it? Most of us have probably seen someone suffering, lingering, or only *existing* without apparent cognition of the world and said to ourselves, "I wouldn't want to live that way. I would want to just go on out." That decision, in our society, is for you and you alone and thus must be made while you can still be the one calling the shots (or pills).

The question of a dying person taking affirmative actions to end his or her life sits at the intersection of so many human concerns: spiritual, social, familial, physical, moral, practical, legal, and even financial. Let's look at four recommendations for those who may be faced with the decision:

Have a mental health assessment.

Aging and illness cause stress. Stress can cause anxiety and depression, and those can be factors in wanting to end one's life at any age. In some cases, these mental and emotional health issues may not be adequately addressed amidst all the immediate physical ones. Don't let that happen. Many antidepressants and anti-anxiety medications and therapies can coexist with whatever physical conditions and treatments you may have. With chronic pain and decreased mobility and a poor prognosis for living much longer, a perfectly rational person may begin to fall into despair to the point of no longer wanting to live and taking affirmative steps to die. But it should not be based on treatable mental health issues, and whatever can improve your sense of well-being in the time you have left is worth trying.

Make sure your decisions are based on sound criteria after investigating alternatives such as enhanced pain management and hospice care.

Everyone has his or her own personal priorities, but choosing to end one's life while there are still opportunities for happiness in it just because your continued existence inconveniences someone else doesn't seem like sound judgement to me. We've heard it many times. 'I don't want to be a burden to anyone. I don't want anyone to have to help me with the toilet. If I can't be productive, I don't want to continue living. If I'm not in my 'right mind' I would rather just go on." None of us would welcome any of those things, but your last days (which may be an extended amount of time) may still hold moments of happiness. One way to better understand the "I don't want to be a burden" argument is to have an honest conversation with your loved ones. Is my present state a debilitating burden to you? Can we still talk, remember, laugh, even if it's all within the confines of one room? Is my income sufficient for my upkeep, instead of causing someone else to literally go hungry? *Or is it more a matter of convenience?*

We are more than our work, our income, our self-sufficiency. Our continued existence is not a matter of someone else's schedule, especially someone for whom we sacrificed, and there could well be resources, such as the respite care benefit in hospice, to give our family a break.

Constant pain can be another factor in the decision. Because of our dystopian opiate epidemic, doctors may be reluctant to prescribe sufficient pain medication, and, sadly, the problem is real. I worked in federal law enforcement for two decades and saw how some families considered having a close relative nearing death a goldmine. Pawpaw's prescription for oxycodone, procured for a $15.00 co-pay with the United Mine Workers retiree health benefits card, could be turned into $2,000 on the street. During her years administering a hospice organization, my wife saw many instances of opiates meant to relieve a dying person's pain stolen by family members for use or resale. Now, in my humble opinion, THOSE are the people who should be really fearing their last breaths. Theft can take many forms, even after the patient is gone.

When I worked for the court, we had a case in which an elderly man lived with his grandchildren in a rural area, and his Social Security and other benefits supplemented the family income. Pawpaw died at home, and we have no reason to believe any foul play was involved. The family was reluctant to lose that income, though, so didn't report the death, instead burying Pawpaw in the crawlspace under the house, wrapped in blankets and complete with his prosthetic leg. "How's your Pawpaw doing?" "Oh, he doesn't get out much anymore." I'll say. Like in many criminal cases, they weren't caught until another family member, cut out from the monthly check income, snitched. "We took good care of Pawpaw. We know this is what he would have wanted," the perpetrators said. That could well be true. But there's that federal crime thingy to think about as well. The photographic evidence submitted as part of the record in that case was not pleasant to see.

If constant pain cannot be sufficiently mitigated, though, the thought of ending one's life may be all but inevitable. We haven't walked in those bed slippers and shouldn't judge. *Yes, I have great pain, even when medicated. Yes, the medication makes me disorientated. But can I still, at times, experience snippets of happiness?* When put on the scale, this may be life's most difficult decision to weigh.

Another poor criterion for ending one's life is arrogance. Edit: that sounds really callous, so let's say *the need to be in control* instead. *I'm no longer calling the shots in this family? Others make decisions for me? I'll show them. I'll go out on my own terms! If I can't have life just the way I want it, darn it, I just won't have it at all. A bonus is that some of my family members might plead with me to not make this decision. I'll show them. SCORE!*

Don't think it doesn't happen. While it may be darkly comforting to think about how various family and associates may react to your demise, remember that: *a.* you may be wrong about them, and *b.* you will get no satisfaction from it, because of that "being dead" situation.

This brings back memories of overhearing adult conversations about end-of-life care in my Appalachian childhood, and my understanding of the medical term *spearmint.* Doctors, while in one way revered, were simultaneously viewed with some disdain, for a few reasons. They were, by the standards of most coalfield families, *rich*, and the idea that "they just keep you coming back to make more money" was prevalent. In those days, "bedside manner" and communicating with patients were not emphasized in medical school (is it significantly better today? I hope so). There was also the belief that doctors kept people alive just so they could continue to bill, or, even worse, to use the patient as a guinea pig to try new (and expensive) treatments to see if they work, no matter the pain or efficacy for the individual. No one wanted that. Hence, "They can't really do nothing for him. They're just spearminting on him. When it's my time to go, don't let them spearmint on me like that." (Get it? If not, it will come to you dreckly, and I say that with all love and affection for my people.)

Consider a patient with ALS as an example. If the disease is rapidly progressing, is it rational to want to end one's life before the inevitable result, perhaps even while still able to independently function to some degree? Even if it's not the decision you would want a loved one to make, the *rationality* of it is hard to deny.

Remember that no matter what you have told everyone and what arrangements you have or have not made, you can always change your mind while you are alert and oriented.

Even at the point that you have taken drugs to end your life, the effects will not likely be immediate, and for some time can be reversed should you request it. Changing one's mind is not cowardly or disappointing yourself or someone else, even a second or third time. It's your right.

If, after all these considerations and preparations and interventions and alternatives have been pursued you come to the decision that you want to take affirmative steps to end your suffering, how is it done? It's not always as simple as one would think.

First, let's clear something up: physician-assisted death is not euthanasia. If a doctor purposely administers a drug that ends someone's life, even if that person asks for the procedure, that is *euthanasia* and is illegal in the United States (think Dr. Kevorkian), though it is legal in some European countries. Even the term *assisted suicide* is problematic because the patient may, indeed, want to continue living but feel the illness has made that no longer tenable. The term *death with dignity*, often used in legal or political circles when considering the practice, implies that some deaths lack it.

But the term physician-assisted death, while not perfect, is as good as we have at present. After in-depth consultation with a terminally ill patient, a physician prescribes life-ending medication which the patient administers to herself or himself. In the past, the drugs would most likely be high doses of barbiturates, either pentobarbital or secobarbital. Those are in short supply and very expensive these days, though, because of controversy over their use in executing prisoners condemned to death, so the prescription may be for high doses of some combination of diazepam, dioxin, morphine, amitriptyline, and propranolol. Physician-assisted death is, as of this writing, legal with various restrictions in California, Colorado, Hawaii, Maine, Montana, New Jersey, New Mexico, Oregon, Vermont, and Washington DC. The general guidelines require that patients:

- Be 18 years of age or older
- Live in the state allowing the procedure
- Be terminally ill (have six months or less to live, as confirmed by at least two doctors)
- Be mentally competent to make their own decisions
- Must make multiple requests, both in writing and in at least one private conversation with the doctor
- Take the medication on their own (source: deathwithdignity.org)

The mental competency requirement means that patients with Alzheimer's disease or other dementia disorders may not be able to make the decision to end their lives with medical assistance.

A doctor is not required, as far as I have been able to ascertain, to be specifically trained or certified in physician-assisted death in order to go through the process and write the prescriptions. There also isn't a comprehensive registry of physicians who will assist, and any doctor may refuse to do so. And (surprise!) neither the service nor the drugs are free. That's the American way! Whether or not your health insurance will pay for them is between you and the company.

If the patient ultimately does choose to take the life-ending drugs, she or he will usually do so either at home or a care facility. There may not be firm statistics on this, but it's estimated that around a third of patients who obtain the prescriptions do not end up administering them to themselves. It serves as a sort of "Plan Z, last-option insurance policy" to have just in case.

A large majority (around 70%, according to a 2018 Gallup poll) of Americans support the right to physician-assisted death. Why, then, is it legal in only nine states and DC? And does that mean it never happens anywhere else? Ah, politics. Remember when the Affordable Care Act was being passed and a certain Alaskan politician eying the Vice Presidency and who really looked like a not-so-carefully-made-up version of Tina Fey ranted about "Death panels," claiming a supposed committee of doctors and/or bureaucrats would decide which patients "deserved" treatment, leaving everyone else to die?

While the desired outcome is to peacefully slip off into sleep and never awaken, there is always the possibility of complications. The sheer volume of drugs, either pills (possibly up to 100 of them, crushed or emptied from capsules and mixed with a sufficient volume of liquid) or in liquid form, that need to be ingested can be daunting for patients who have trouble swallowing, and can cause stomach upset. Vomiting could reduce the drugs to an ineffective level, so an antiemetic is taken beforehand. Since that will eventually wear off, everything must be ingested in a set amount of time. Patients who have gastric absorption problems may also not get a sufficient does of drugs despite getting them all down.

Even when everything works, how long the drugs take to bring about death is unpredictable. It could be an hour. It could be six or longer. During that time, instead of sleeping peacefully, there is the possibility of gasping and choking, sphincters releasing, and other unpleasant-to-think-about death throes occurrences.

I am not purposely trying to upset or sway anyone's decision by describing what can happen, but just be aware that the "peacefully drifting off" scenario we picture from scenes in movies, while possible, is in no way guaranteed. And it could well be that a terminally ill patient may not be able to prepare all these things alone or choose to *be* alone when dying. So, while it may be known as physician-assisted death, that's a misnomer in a way. Yes, Doc did the paperwork, but Doc isn't there, so it falls on Bubba and Sally to be in the room helping their dad, squeezing capsules and mixing white powder with corn syrup and wondering how much was lost when Pappy threw up just a little bit.

What if you have made the rational decision to seek medical aid in dying, but you don't live in one of the states that allow it? One option is to move to a state that does and go through the consultation process with a doctor there, which can be an onerous and expensive requirement for someone very ill. Most states with medical aid in dying laws do require residency. (Oregon and Vermont may be exceptions in some cases but consult professionals in those states about your individual circumstances before considering making arrangements. Some who are able travel more extensively and have the means go to countries with broader life-ending assistance laws and infrastructure in place, such as Canada, Belgium, the Netherlands, Luxembourg, or Switzerland).

Then, after the meds are prescribed, do you stay in that state while contemplating your final decision or move back home? If you stay, pre-plan with a local mortuary how to have your remains transported back to your home state. The option of taking the drugs back home isn't as simple as it sounds. If you take life-ending drugs in a state without laws that address the practice, your death may be ruled a suicide, which could affect life insurance payouts and other benefits. There are many potential complications to consider.

If you choose to not take the drugs, they, like all controlled substance prescriptions, must be disposed of in whatever legal manner mandated by the local jurisdiction. Hospice care workers (many patients who choose life-ending drugs receive the service), should be able to assist with that. One thing you *don't* do is take the drugs in a public place, as many of the laws specifically note that your estate will be liable for any expense incurred by local services. So, as tempting as taking your last breath sitting by the fireplace at your favorite Cracker Barrel restaurant may be, it's not a good idea.

If moving to another state isn't possible or desirable, what then? You may choose to revert to the *Passively allow the process to take its course* option we discussed earlier. You can stop taking meds (other than those for pain and anxiety) and other treatments. Demise can be hastened by also voluntarily choosing to stop eating and drinking, a prospect unlikely to sound palatable to any of us today, but may be more so for someone, for instance, who receives nutrition and hydration through a tube, or who is in such pain that she or he receives no pleasure from these activities and hunger and thirst are numbed.

As death nears, stronger pain management may be needed to relieve what are known as *refractory symptoms*, perhaps to the point of patient unconsciousness. Some may think this level of "palliative sedation" hastens death, but in some circumstances the affect may be just the opposite. For example, if a patient is receiving a maximum flow of oxygen but continues respiratory distress, morphine may relieve it and prolong the dying process instead of shortening it.

We have probably all heard grieving but uninformed family members say things like "they killed Pawpaw by keeping him so doped up." Pawpaw's fighting and thrashing and being in tremendous pain instead of being "doped up" could actually shorten his life instead of lengthening it, in addition to being cruel. Yes, too much morphine near death can hasten it, but in some circumstances so can too little, and leave your loved one in misery. There's my opinion.

The sad truth is that, facing pain and a terminal diagnosis, a sizable number of people each year choose actual suicide. I have known more than one personally. Were medically assisted hastening of the inevitable more available and socially acceptable, perhaps there would be fewer. We don't really know what that number is, because some hasten their death through means not obvious enough to be classified as suicide. Squirreling away enough morphine or other opiate over time little by little so it isn't missed and then deliberately taking it all at once may be determined as a dosing error or not even thoroughly investigated for a terminal patient.

One option you *don't* have is to mandate medically assisted death in your advance directive, as it cannot be legally honored. It is a decision that must be made while you are alert and oriented and able to participate in the act.

How do you decide? No one can answer for you, but knowing what questions to ask can help. My friends at Compassion in Dying, a nonprofit organization in London, England have developed one of the most striking and useful documents I have found in my research, and they have given me permission to share it with you (thanks for your help, Jennifer Noel!). Titled I WANT TO KNOW, this checklist of questions to ask and options to consider if you are given a terminal diagnosis is comprehensive, straight forward, and easy to use (with slight modifications for an American audience)

IF GIVEN A TERMINAL DIAGNOSIS, I WANT TO KNOW:

What does my diagnosis mean and what can I expect?

What is my outlook for the future, as you see it? How was the diagnosis made? Might my diagnosis change? How advanced is my illness?

What are the symptoms I am likely to experience, both now and as my illness progresses?

What kind of changes will I have to make in my work, family life, sex life, and leisure time?

My other thoughts and questions:

Will I get the support I need?

Where will I be cared for?

Who will be part of my healthcare team? Will there be different people involved?

Will I need any equipment in my home as my condition progresses?

What support is available to help me and my family? Who

should I contact if things get worse? Can my family members be involved in decisions?

How long have I got?

How long am I likely to live for? Am I likely to die from this illness?

What will happen when I am dying?

What will happen to me at the very end? How will I die? Will I be conscious at the end? Will I be in pain?

My other thoughts and questions:

My priority is...

A. To live as long as possible?

What treatments will enable me to live as long as possible? Can you slow down the progression of my illness?

B. To have a good quality of life?

Would your recommendation change if I told you that my priority is having a good quality of life, so, living as normally as possible for as long as possible?

How will this illness affect my quality of life?

I like to (things you most enjoy and want to be able to do):

How can I ensure I get to do these things for as long as possible?

What are the best things I can do to stay as healthy as possible?

I do not want to swap a bad situation for something worse. Could this treatment make me feel worse than my illness already makes me feel?

Treatment decisions:

What are my treatment options?

What are my treatment options? Can you explain the benefits and things I should consider for each one?

Are there other ways to treat my illness? Do I need more than one sort of treatment?

Is my decision urgent or can I take more time to think about it? What will happen if the treatment is delayed?

What will the treatment be like? How long will it take?

If the treatment you are suggesting does not work,

or the side effects are bad, what are the other options?

Where will I have this treatment? Will it be in hospital? How long will I be in there?

My other thoughts and questions:

What will this treatment do?

What is the aim of this treatment? Will it cure the illness, or will it just help my symptoms or slow the illness down?

Are there any risks with this treatment? Is there any chance that this treatment will make me worse? How will I know if the treatment is working?

How many people in my situation benefit from this treatment?

Are there side effects?

Are there any side effects? If there are side effects, what are they like, and can anything be done about them?

If I find the side effects unacceptable, can I stop the treatment?

Not having treatment:

What will happen if I choose not to have treatment? What is the natural course of my illness if left untreated?

After treatment:

How will I feel after the treatment? How long will it take after treatment to recover? What will my life be like during and after the treatment?

I like to (things you most enjoy and want to be able to do):

Will I be able to do these things after this treatment?

Having tests:

What will the results of this test tell me?

How will the result affect your recommendation for my treatment?

How will this test help me decide about treatment?

My religion and spiritual beliefs:

How can I access spiritual support?

How can I be supported to ensure any rituals important to me are honored?

How can I be referred to a representative of my faith or a Chaplain?

My other thoughts and questions:

Things to find out about:

Where can I get counselling?

Are there any support groups for me and/or my care giver?

What benefits am I entitled to?

What support is available at home, for example nursing, help with washing and dressing, and help with shopping?

Will I need practical living aids and equipment, and how can I arrange this?

Who can I call if I am worried or my health changes?

I live on my own, so do I need a personal alarm to alert people if I fall or am in trouble?

Am I entitled to a handicapped placard?

My other thoughts and questions:

Some of the questions are impossible to answer definitively, of course. They require you to set your own priorities. Everyone in the medical profession is busy but be persistent until you are satisfied your questions have been answered to the best of their ability. Even then, your decisions will not likely be easy ones. Remember you can always change them, until you can't. In that regard, it is like buying new carpet, but with even higher stakes.

Have you, or should you, make provisions for organ donation? It certainly saves lives, and there is a severe shortage of all types. According to the University of Pennsylvania Health System, it is estimated that approximately 17 people die each day waiting for an organ to become available for transplant. Transplants are not like replacing car parts with new OEM pieces. It is often a constant struggle to avoid rejection, and a significant number simply fail. Kidneys are the most transplanted organ, and those recipients have the longest average post-transplant lifespan (20+ years). Lung recipients average less than half that (9.28 years).

It's more complicated than it sounds, though. It's easy to think, "Hey, I don't need those things anymore, so why not put them to good use?" and that is certainly valid. Keep in mind that, depending on your age and physical condition, there may simply not be much left worth harvesting. Even if your organs do not meet the criteria, sections of skin and bone donated for grafts may make a tremendous difference in someone's life. Most bodies have something of value.

That said, many people, even those who have the organ donor designation on their driver's license, may not fully understand what happens as a result. We may have the image of our dramatic and touching media-driven death scene, then being whisked into surgery to remove the useful bits, but that's not how it often happens. Every minute an organ is without oxygenated blood flow reduces that organ's viability, so our discussion above of the greyish definition of death, either medical or legal, is important. When patients are pronounced dead by neurological criteria, their hearts may still be beating, and removing the body from a ventilator to await the pulse's cessation may not be the best practice for successful transplants.

In the words of Dr. Robert M. Sade of The Medical University of South Carolina, "A brain dead individual who is warm and pink with heart beating and lungs ventilating is just as dead, legally, as an individual whose body has turned cold after the heart has permanently stopped beating... The patient is brought to the operating room, life support is withdrawn, and when the heart stops after a few minutes to an hour without ventilation or other support, the physician observes the patient for a few minutes to ensure that the heart does not start beating again spontaneously. If there continues to be no circulation for 2–5 minutes, the physician pronounces the patient dead. At this point, the transplant team enters the operating room and removes organs, usually the kidneys and liver, from the now dead patient." (42)

Remember the accepted definition of death: An individual who has sustained EITHER (1) irreversible cessation of circulatory and respiratory functions, OR (2) irreversible cessation of all functions of the entire brain, including the brain stem, is dead. A determination of death must be made in accordance with accepted medical standards. So, a patient can be declared dead under this definition and still have a beating heart and still be oxygenating his or her organs with the aid of a ventilator or, for a time, even spontaneously. In the scenario described by Dr. Sade, the patient's pulse could (not that it SHOULD), in many cases, be restored by immediate cardiopulmonary resuscitation and the ventilator reconnected. So, was that technically irreversible?

If you intend to be an organ donor, let your loved ones know that they may be given the chance to say their final goodbyes when you are still "warm and pink with heart beating and lungs ventilating." Without being prepared, that could cause someone subconsciously still clinging to false hope for recovery even more distress.

My first wife's death was the only one in which I have been the decision maker, and I hope it is the last. I did not choose organ donation for her. Jennifer's pulse and unaided breathing continued for about an hour after the ventilator was removed. At least I think it was that long, or maybe a bit longer. Although I am OCD about time and detail, the whole thing is compressed in my memory, fuzzy like I was on the outside looking in, so I don't know for sure.

Can your family override your informed directive to donate your organs? In most cases, no. Can your next of kin allow donation even if you have not signed consent yourself? In most cases, yes. Does it affect whether you can have an open-casket funeral? No.

What in our lives has ever been simple? It should come as no surprise that neither is death. While you should think about it and make all the applicable decisions and directives, don't dwell on it. Go out and enjoy every minute…as soon as you have all your decisions made and your paperwork in order.

WHAT HAPPENS TO YOUR BODY NEXT?

That depends on the circumstances and what arrangements you have made or, instead, left for someone else to make. It also depends on where you die, and that has been changing. Up until the second part of the 1900s, most people died at home. Then it shifted to most people dying in hospitals. In 2017, though, it shifted again, when non-hospital deaths outnumbered hospital deaths for the first time in more than half a century, according to a *New England Journal of Medicine* study quoted by Reuters (December 11, 2019). Home hospice care is one of the primary reasons for the shift.

The article contains an eyebrow-raising quote from Dr. Haider Warraich, Associate Director of the Heart Failure Program in the Boston, Virginia Healthcare System, and coauthor of the study along with Dr. Sarah Cross of the Duke University Sanford School of Public Policy. *"More people dying at home is good news,"* he said. How's that for an example of the importance of context?

If you are receiving hospice care, a plan for what happens when you die is part of the process. As death draws nearer, the hospice nurse will likely visit more frequently, and come to the home when death is imminent. She or he will be able to complete the paperwork necessary for a death certificate and contact the mortuary or crematorium of your choice. The nurse may also clean the body if needed and make sure it is in a prone position before rigor mortis begins to set in.

If you are not receiving hospice care and choose to die at home, it is even more important to have a plan in place. Exactly what you need to have your family do may depend on local regulations. Work with your doctor or funeral director to develop a step-by-step list, and make sure your caregivers understand it. Of course, that assumes your death isn't sudden and unexpected, but making sure all your directives are in place and loved ones know what/where they are (assembled with other important documents in *The Book of the Still Living* as opposed to the anciently famous *Book of the Dead*) no matter how hale and hearty you are is still important.

For the almost half of us who will die in a hospital, it's common for hospital staff to allow our loved ones a short time with our body in the hospital room before it is moved to the hospital morgue, where it will be stored until taken to the mortuary or crematorium of the family's choice. When the body arrives at a mortuary, it will be cleaned if needed and refrigerated until prepared for the disposition.

Whether or not that includes embalming is usually a choice, except in a few states and even then only under specific circumstances, such as transportation across state lines. Morticians may want you to assume it's for the best because it's profitable for them, and the process does lengthen the amount of time the body can remain unrefrigerated (for viewing and services in most cases) before being buried. If the body is embalmed, suction is applied to one of the veins and the blood is drained. A solution of formaldehyde and water is injected into a main artery; fluid is drawn from the abdominal cavity with a long needle and replaced with a preservative. The organs are not removed.

When a body is to be cremated, it is, like Haulover Beach, "clothing optional." A simple sheet is used, unless the family requests the deceased be dressed, such as when cremation follows a viewing. More often, the cremation takes place first and a memorial service, with the urn in attendance, occurs later. Even then, the clothing must be fully combustible. The body is placed into a wooden or strong paper container after jewelry is removed. Pacemakers also must go, of course, because they contain batteries. Other metal objects such as artificial joints and amalgam fillings stay, but, if sizable, will be removed from the remains after cremation.

The container is rolled into a specially designed cremation chamber called a *retort* (though a witty comeback is most unlikely). The temperature can reach 2,000 degrees, and the process take 2-3 hours depending on the equipment and the deceased's size. What's left is referred to as ashes but is mostly bone fragments since everything else is gasified by the extreme heat and released through the chimney. After cremation and cooling down, the remains, typically weighing 3-9 pounds, are often processed by grinding the fragments into a finer powder form and placed into a container.

Two Deaths – A Personal Story

By our age, most of us have experienced the death of someone close to us. The first I remember, in 1965, was of my paternal grandmother, who had been born during the waning years of the 19th century. First, that is, unless you count my earliest clear memory, when I was four and a half: my aunt and my Mom and I were at the post office in Beaver, West Virginia picking up the mail before going Christmas shopping. The post mistress came to the window and cried, "They've shot the president, in Dallas!" I probably remember it so well because of how it affected my Mom and aunt. A few days later, the large family who were our closest farm neighbors came into our living room and sat on the floor to watch President Kennedy's funeral, because they didn't have a television set. Some pundits define a Baby Boomer by whether you have a memory of President Kennedy's assassination, no matter how young you were at the time.

But, back to the other deaths that affected me: Grandma had been in the hospital for a long while recovering from a cholecystectomy, which required an extended hospital stay back then. She never did well afterwards and then had a stroke. My parents wouldn't let me see her in the casket, believing a 6 ½ year old wasn't mature enough to do so. I missed grandma, who was quite nice, and saw my father suffer bouts of depression after losing her. My paternal grandfather, who I remember as being less nice, died while I was in junior high school after lingering in the hospital for more than a week. Sad, but expected.

When I was in the ninth grade, though, one of my school chums died of Reye's Syndrome. He had the flu, and we did not yet know that giving aspirin to youngsters in such situations could lead to this often-fatal neurological disease. Afterwards, my father found me sitting in a dark room playing a record of a song sung at my buddy's funeral and told me to be a man and snap out of it. A cascade of other grandparents and aunts and uncles dying followed as I became an adult. My maternal grandfather had the best of it. He was driving along the single-lane blacktopped road from the farm to go out for a haircut. That had to be a social visit since he was bald as an egg and had been since they stopped making Packards. A neighbor saw grandpa's Chevy Malibu in the ditch with the back wheels still slowly spinning and came out to see what was wrong. Grandpa was slumped on the steering wheel, dead. No needles, no hospital, no time to even put the car in park.

But the two death experiences that affected me most came in unexpectedly quick succession when I was in my late 40s. My father was a retired coal miner, and had Black Lung Disease, silicosis, and COPD. Though he had stopped around age 70, he had been a smoker since he was an early teen, so had probably logged more than a half century of Lucky Strikes, Kents, and Kools. One day he called me into the spare bedroom at his house and told me his doctor had found "something" in his lung and there wasn't "really anything they can do about it." He died of lung cancer less than a year later.

It wasn't a *good* year. While Dad looked fine that day, his decline was rapid. He began to lose weight. He was administered a new drug for lung cancer, called Tarciva, but his insurance kept battling over whether to pay for it. In the end, it didn't matter. He lost his appetite, had the energy to do little more than sit on the sofa, and the formerly almost-chubby Pawpaw beloved by my daughters transformed into an ashen skeleton. We all felt so bad for him. That Christmas, the one we all knew would be his last, we took a family group photo, the last one with us all together before the lens.

The part I still have trouble fully understanding came just a few months before he died. He developed an intestinal blockage that caused him suffering and put him into the hospital. The surgeon said it was probably a rapid spread of cancer, and, if that were the case, death would come quickly. The only way to make sure was to operate, which my emaciated father may not survive. While stating the options as he was obligated to do, the surgeon clearly did not want to do operate, but instead administer "comfort care" to make sure Dad passed on peacefully.

At this point, Dad was cogent and could make his own decisions. He was in such misery and distress, his time left was obviously so short, the pain and ultimate futility of the surgery so sure and his quality of life was so poor, that I thought the choice was obvious: It was time to go.

But that's not at all what he decided. I felt it was a horrible choice, but there with my mother, brother, and daughter, I could not bring myself to say, "Dad, let's talk about this and what's likely to happen, and make sure this is what you really want." No one else did either, and I don't even know if they were thinking it. Dad wanted to live, and Mom wanted him to as well. We all did. But I was not brave enough to get them to think about the definition of just what *live* meant in his condition.

The blockage turned out not to be aggressive cancer, and Dad lived another few months while continuing to waste away in pain and sadness. He refused hospice care, saying he didn't want to die at home because Mom would think about him lying there dead every time she went into the bedroom. So it was that he spent several of his final days in the hospital. The last words he said to me that I could understand over the pumping CPAP were "Y'all don't fight." The next evening, he was unconscious and moved to a hospice facility, where he died the following morning without having regained consciousness.

We had almost a year to prepare for Dad's death. Remember that Christmas photo I mentioned? Little did I know.

About seven months later, we had one of our frequent ice storms in the mountains of southern West Virginia. School was called off for the day, but the federal court wasn't closed and I went on to work, in our main office more than 50 miles away. My wife, a middle school teacher, found some trash she wanted to take out, slipped on the ice, and broke her leg. She had her cell phone with her (thankfully) and called for an ambulance. There being a lack of orthopedic surgeons in our area, she ended up in a hospital more than a hundred miles from home. The surgery went well, we were told, and I spent a lot of time over the next couple of days reading by her bedside while she was groggy.

In the evening, I went into the bath of her hospital room to shower. When I turned the water off, I heard commotion in the room, so I quickly pulled on my clothes and opened the door. Several staff members were frantically doing things around her bed, and I was unceremoniously pushed out into the hallway. I heard the distinctive whine of an AED charging. It turned out that, after 20+ years of marriage and two children, my last words to Jennifer Lynn Thompson Kuhn that I know she could hear were "I'm going in to take a shower."

Time seemed compressed. A social worker and a chaplain took me to a quiet area and "explained" that something terrible had happened and my wife had gone into cardiac arrest. While she had been revived by restarting her heart, her brain had been without oxygen for so long that she had no higher brain activity and was being kept alive by a ventilator. When they were allowed to take me back in to see her, it was plain to me that she was gone, despite air being pumped in and out of her lungs. Over the next three days, I sat by her side. Occasionally, she would open her eyes for a few seconds, then close them again. There was never a response to pinpricks to her feet and no upper brain activity registered in scans.

I called my daughters to have them drive a hundred miles to say goodbye to their mother. I sent them home after two days. By that time, doctors were suggesting I give consent to remove the ventilator and IV hydration. I talked with the hospital's Catholic chaplain, and he agreed that would be the right decision...after making a derogatory joke about Hillary Clinton. I suppose he felt that was safe to do because I was a white Catholic male in West Virginia. He seemed rather embarrassed that it didn't offer comic relief to my distress. Jerk.

Not long afterward, I was surprised when the nun from our parish, a friend and by no means young, walked in, having heard what was happening and driving a hundred miles in the winter to be with us. She had with her a young doctor who, as a boy, had sat with his family in a pew near us each Sunday. He examined her and told me with both gentleness and appreciated frankness that she had very little time left. As it turned out, he was correct, and Jennifer died with me holding one hand and Sister Janice the other, about ten minutes later. She gasped a bit and stopped breathing. She was 50.

Dad's death was anticipated, and, frankly, welcomed given the state of his existence. Jennifer's was not. Dad had signed a Do Not Resuscitate order as part of his advance directive package. Jennifer had not. It is not an easy thing to write about my father and the mother of my children, but, under their circumstances, they both lived longer than they should, one by months and one by days. Both spent a few days "in a coma" as laypeople sometimes call it.

During that time, a great deal of effort and money were expended essentially keeping two disintegrating corpses just within the legal parameters of "life." Multiply those resources by how many? Approximately 3.37 million Americans die each year. Ridiculously futile and unnecessary (and even cruel, at times) "treatment" is not administered in all those deaths but think of the number of times it does happen. During the time my father and my wife's bodies were kept "alive," people went to work sick and spread their illnesses to everyone around them because they couldn't afford medical care or a day to stay home. Children went unvaccinated, untreated diabetes ravaged hearts and kidneys, people with mental illness shivered on the streets, and old people developed bed sores from inattention. Something isn't quite right.

How can we avoid a similar fate for ourselves? Tie up all the advance directive loose ends possible, communicate with your family, and then hope for the best. Believing you can do more, that you can *assure* your control of how your life ends, is, I am afraid, wishful thinking. Do your best, then live your life.

THE FINAL GREAT GIFT

If everything you have read above doesn't convince you of the need to have directives in place, I don't know what will. Most everyone agrees, I think, but only about a third of adults have done it, a statistic that is shocking, disappointing, and sad. (43) There is practically no plausible argument against it, so why don't we do it? Like many other things, it comes down to a quote often attributed to Buddha but actually comes from Jack Kornfield's lovely interpretation of Buddhist philosophy, *Buddha's Little Instruction Book* (Bantam Books, May 1, 1994): "The trouble is, you think you have time."

That simple statement can apply to almost everything we have discussed in this book, and everything else we haven't discussed, for that matter. I hope it sticks in your mind like a movie popcorn hull sticks between your molars.

Having your bureaucratic affairs in order will help give you peace of mind. As to your loved ones, I can tell you firsthand what it is like to deal with a death with no directives or other planning documents in place. It compounds the pain of loss. Please do not foist those decisions upon anyone else at what could be one of the most difficult times of their lives.

Legal documents: The most important is the Advance Healthcare Directive, popularized some years ago with the warm and fuzzy name Living Will. It tells healthcare professionals what kind of treatment and intervention you want if you are not able to make and communicate such decisions at the time. This includes both emergency and longer-term treatments and under what circumstances the directive is to apply. Let's make something very,

very clear: Regardless of what directive you have in place, if you can make and communicate your own wishes at any time during medical treatment, those supersede any written directive. You are not giving up the right to make your own decisions later.

Hey, I found a Living Will form and printed it off and signed it, so I'm good to go, right? It may not be so simple. Many forms, especially older ones, may simply address "no heroic measures be taken" or some such nebulous language. Some new ones are better, including specific directives on such things as

- Determining if and when cardiopulmonary resuscitation (CPR) or using a defibrillator to restart your heart if it has stopped beating should be administered.
- Whether or not a ventilator should be used to take over your respiration if you're unable to breathe on your own. If so, for how long and under what circumstances?
- If unable to take nutrition while unconscious, do you want tube feeding to supply your body with nutrients and fluids intravenously and/or via a tube inserted into your stomach. If so, for how long and under what circumstances?
- Do you wish to have kidney dialysis to remove waste from your blood and manage fluid levels if your kidneys no longer function? If so, for how long and under what circumstances?
- If you are near the end of life, do you want aggressive antibiotics or antiviral medications or would you rather let infections run their course?
- Do you wish to be an organ doner?

The other important document concerning your treatment is a medical power of attorney, or *durable power of attorney for healthcare.* It appoints another person, called a proxy, to make healthcare decisions for you if you are unable to do so for yourself. It is important that the person you name is familiar with your wishes. But be fully prepared that this may require something we apparently go to great lengths to avoid: having a conversation with our loved ones about, you know, *it.* And I don't mean sex this time.

Do you need both? You may. Since a Living Will is usually very general, it may not cover the myriad specific decisions that are often required even if someone is unable to make and communicate those decisions themselves. That's an important thing to remember: this document doesn't assume your imminent death, but instead covers any time you are unable to make and communicate your own decisions, and it does not come into effect unless that happens.

What happens if the two conflict? It can certainly happen. Here's a scenario: You have a Living Will specifying you do not want to be connected to a ventilator. That may be a valid choice for you, perhaps influenced by the experience of seeing a loved one without a directive lying as essentially a corpse with air being pushed in an out of its lungs. Most of us want to avoid that. But think about those dark days of the COVID pandemic: there are lots of people walking around today who survived the disease even though they were unconscious for a time with a ventilator being used without their knowledge or express consent. In such a case, one's appointed proxy, in consultation with the doctor, may decide those are not the circumstances you anticipated when signing the Living Will and make a different decision. What happens then?

It depends. State laws vary on the matter, and many are silent on it. Some would look to the dates on which the two documents were signed, while others could only settle the matter in court. I wish I had a better answer. If nothing else, this reaffirms the importance of being specific as you can in the documents, having in-depth conversations with your proxy, and consulting a local lawyer instead of solely relying on a catch-all generic document found on the internet (which is still better than having nothing, though).

Disposition arrangements: I use this term instead of funeral arrangements here because you may not want a funeral, and that's your right. But whatever is left, be it a body or ashes, must go somewhere. You may not really care (you will, after all, be dead), but it is kindness to relieve anyone left behind from having to make those decisions. There are some wonderful folks in the funeral industry, but there are also many who are willing to squeeze maximum profit from bereaved families at a vulnerable time. Pre-planning (is there another kind?) can avoid that happening.

THE BOOK OF THE STILL LIVING

While this former high school science teacher has given you lots of information and "best practices" gleaned from trusted sources, there haven't been many specific homework assignments until this chapter. Okay, I made some strong suggestions in Chapter 1, but that wasn't homework, per se. That is about to change.

Go to your local discount store (one that favors yellow bags is such a presence in my native state of West Virginia that they can be used as a measure of distance. "After you turn left on Rt. 219 in Lewisburg, go two Dollar Generals and then look for what used to be an Exxon station on the right.") and spend about ten bucks on a binder, a package of notebook paper, some tabs, a hole punch, and a smoothly-writing gel pen. That small investment is the beginning of a project that will become a gift without price for your family and as well as yourself.

In case you have failed to get the idea yet, you are going to die. I hope it's a long time from now, after you have had the chance to recommend this book to everyone you know and buy lots of them as gifts, but *it's going to happen*. I also hope you have time to settle your affairs and make all your amends and put everything in order before gently drifting off to join your ancestors. Sometimes that happens, but there is certainly no guarantee.

As glum an exercise as it may be, consider this question: if I have a heart attack and die unexpectedly at 2:00 AM tomorrow, exactly what will take place among my loved ones? Will they know what to do? Will they be able to access all the necessary information in the first hours, days, month, year? While we all need to accept the fact that we can't control things from the grave, shouldn't our instructions and arrangements be spelled out as clearly as we can? What can we do now to make following those arrangements less burdensome and thus more likely to be followed?

Then, on a more personal note, what things about yourself do you want them to know, but just haven't been shared for one reason or another? Or, if they have been shared, do you want to make sure will be remembered and available for your later descendants who will never even meet you?

Finally, before going to bed that ill-fated final night, how much time did you waste not being able to find information that is important, but only occasionally needed to access? And how much time do you spend chatting with old friends and family members about your shared experiences?

The answers to those questions could fill a book. *The Book of the Still Living.* Tell your family what you are doing. Show them the book so they will know what it looks like and tell them who will have access to it. Let them know at least generally what it contains, and how it will help them do what needs to be done when you are no longer around to do it yourself.

I prefer a loose-leaf binder so pages can be discarded and added at will. Use tabs or cover pages and arrange it in a "first things first" manner. It will be one of the most personal and individual documents you have ever produced and an ongoing project for as long as you are still, ah, *going on*. Start with the sections described below and then give serious thought to what more you want to add for posterity.

Medical Directives and Powers of Attorney

We have already discussed the importance of these documents elsewhere. Copies can be added using the hole punch. Make sure you change the documents out whenever you make revisions. Here you should also specify things like your desire for Anointing of the Sick or other spiritual requests you may be incapable of making when they are required, and people who should be contacted about your condition should you become unable contact them yourself. This section is mainly for use when death may be imminent, and you are no longer making and communicating your own decisions.

Final arrangements

If you have done pre-planning with a mortuary, include a copy of the agreement and the deed to cemetery plots if applicable. Add any burial insurance information. If there are certain clothes, flowers, songs, pallbearers, refreshments, clergy, or anything else you desire, list them in detail. Sometimes these are already on file if you have pre-planned, but it never hurts to repeat them, so everyone knows. I have heard several people over the years say things like "I don't want any kind of service whatsoever. I don't even want anyone to know I'm dead" or "I want a big party!" Perhaps you have, by your own standards, good cause for wanting what you want. But keep in mind you won't be there to see anyone's reactions or hear what they say or sample the meal put together by the Bereavement Committee. If you choose to be considerate to those you leave behind, ask, "What is likely to bring them the most comfort?" using your own experiences of what was or wasn't comforting when you suffered a loss as a guide. Whatever you choose, someone must pay for it. Not everything item can be paid in advance, so address what funds should be used for the rest. Want a bagpiper, for instance? They aren't that easy to find in some places, so give contact info.

Speaking of which, I think this is a good place to add bit of levity to this ponderous subject. Here is a passage from one of my books, *Mountain Mysts: Myths and Fantasies of the Appalachians* (Headline Books, November 2015), relating a conversation between two high school buddies riding around on a Saturday:

"Funny thing, about bagpipes. There're lots of people who say they want them at their funeral, but never listen to them while they are alive. So, they only want to be around them when they can't hear them. But my aunt, she's a nurse's aide in Fairmont, told about an old guy who really loved them though. He was dying in the hospital and didn't have any family at all, but she promised she would make sure he had bagpipes when he was buried. She is just that kind of person."

"I wish you were that kind of person," Walsh said.

"You mean, always wanting to help people, like my aunt?" Altruism, even as a suggestion to someone else, sounded strange coming from Walsh.

"No, like the old guy. Dying," Walsh smirked.

I didn't acknowledge it. "So, she finds out where the old guy was going to be buried, way out in the country somewhere, and hires a bagpiper to play at the graveside. She didn't give him very good directions. She's nice, but a little scatterbrained."

"So you get that pretty natural, I guess." Walsh was quick with that reply.

"Anyway, that bagpiper was all decked out in his kiltie and such, driving out in the country to find the burying, and got lost. Finally, he saw just two guys up on the hill with shovels and said, "Shoot, I've missed it already.' But he's determined the old guy would get what he wanted, plus he was making $25 on the deal, so he screeched up, jumped out, played *Amazing Grace*, and drove off. Mission accomplished. One of the guys with a shovel started to tear up, and said 'Jim Bob, that was the most beautiful thing I've ever seen.' And do you know what Jim Bob said?"

"I'm sure as hell not going to ask for it. I know you're going to tell me anyway." Walsh was right, of course.

"Old Jim Bob dabbed his eyes with his teary bandanna and said 'Sure 'nuff, Eugene, and I've never seen anybody have that kind of respect for a new septic tank before.'"

Your will

Since your executed copy is in a safe or deposit box or with your lawyer, this is likely to be a photocopy. After the official document, delineate all those small things that aren't important enough to put in the will, but that you would like to see go to specific people or organizations, along with any history or explanation why the items are meaningful. We have already talked about the common-sense move of giving those things to loved ones while you can do it and explain it yourself, but you can't do that with everything, or your house would be as empty and uncomfortable as your long-ago collage flat. Keep in mind these instructions will not have the force of law like your will, so all the important stuff should go into that document.

Example: I would like one each of the two Jadeite Fire King C-handle Restaurant Ware coffee mugs in the kitchen cupboard to go to Ashley and Chelsey. Your grandfather drank coffee from them almost every day of his life. What he didn't often mention is that he stole them when he was a teenager from the Skyline Drive In in Oak Hill, West Virginia. This was the same drive-in where, early on New Year's morning 1953, a young driver wheeled a Cadillac in, used the restroom, and checked on his passenger in the back seat. His passenger was country star Hank Williams, and he was dead. Ironically, Hank's body was processed at Tyree Funeral Home, the *same one our family (including Dad) has used for generations. I see similar mugs on eBay for around $40 sometimes, but these are pretty scratched up. Occasionally, I have a cup of coffee from one of them and remember eating breakfast with Dad and how he would drown his pancakes in Karo syrup. I want my grandson to have the battered old Roosevelt for President button in my nightstand drawer. It's not worth hardly anything in that condition, but it came from my grandfather. -Male*

It's easy to figure out who that particular male is, I know. Be as rambling and wordy as you want. There will be plenty of time for brevity and conciseness and sleep after you're dead. In other words, use the opportunity to pass down family history…also known as love.

Your financial/bureaucratic information

You have many things on autopilot, such as monthly bill payments and deposits and withdrawals, etc. Every single one of them will eventually need some type of attention when you are no longer either a payor or payee.

In today's world, that means account numbers, usernames, and passwords.

Those are the bane of my existence, and I am probably not alone. You can hardly order a 12-pack of easily biodegradable RV toilet rolls without setting up an account. Every subscription, every device, every marketplace, every organization, and every service challenge us. "Halt! Who goes there?" "Um…for you, I'm not sure if I am my email address or my initials with a couple of symbols or something else. And that's before I even get to the password. So, never mind. I'll just be on my way." Try to calculate just how many usernames and passwords are out there for you right now, and your estimate will likely fall short.

A 2023 study commissioned by NordPass found the average number of passwords per person is right around one hundred. That's 25% increase over 2020, and it's probably overly optimistic to think the pace will slow. The computer security company Norton tells us the overall quality of our password security is dismal. *123456. Qwerty. Password.* Gasp! I have just revealed three of the most common passwords, right here for the world to see.

No matter if it is your bank or frequent flyer or credit card or mobile phone or Netflix accounts or your Social Security or Thrift Savings Plan portal, the appointed person you trust to settle your affairs will benefit from access to those when you die, and not having them will complicate things. But, obviously, the level of trust must be absolute. That means it will be important to keep your *Book of the Still Living* secure until it's needed and have a plan to keep it that way and specific steps for the right person to access it. In fact, you may find it necessary to do two volumes, one with more restricted access.

Committing all this information to writing will serve a dual purpose because chances are you can't remember all your usernames and passwords right now (who could?), and don't keep an updated comprehensive list of them. Whenever you must log in to an account (something as simple as an electricity or WIFI outage or getting a new device can cause your computer to lose your saved passwords), you may try the phrase you *just know* is correct enough times that you get locked out. Or you rummage through drawers to find that crinkled list with bad handwriting (is that a 0 or a O?) you thought was current amidst several desiccated packets of Taco Bell mild sauce and plastic cutlery. This will be a difficult and time-consuming task, but you will then have the information for yourself all in one place as well as for your left-behinds.

Don't forget safe combinations and where lockbox and safe deposit box and desk keys can be found. Go to any antique store and you will find beautiful old desks with chunks of walnut or oak out of them where locked drawers were pried open. If you are a gun and/or tool chest person, remember those keys and combinations.

Now for the bureaucracy part: Medical and insurance policy account numbers, car VINs, where land and car titles can be found, investment account numbers, death certificate of a deceased spouse, passport numbers, monthly utility account numbers, and contact information for family, friends, financial planners, and anyone else who may need to be contacted or be helpful to those handling your affairs. Note that you may have more insurance policies than you even realize, because sometimes small ones come free with bank accounts or organizational memberships.

So much information! The task may seem so overwhelming that you don't want to tackle it, or start and then give up. Do a little each day. As you use a password or account number or key or pay a bill, put it on the list, and be sure to update it whenever something changes or is added. Go to your phone or computer contact list and print it out or copy it. Include your Christmas card address list if you have one. All the time you spend looking for these items can be avoided if they are in one convenient place. *The Book of the Still Living* will become a welcome aid well before your demise, so putting forth the considerable effort to write it is not purely altruistic.

Your story, or What you want to leave behind that isn't stuff

Over the years, I have made *Books of the Still Living* containing only this section for four older women, including my mother. When I suggested writing about themselves, they all had the same response. *No one would be interested in anything about me. I can't write well, and I can't remember things.* Because the hardest part of any writing assignment is getting started, I started it for them, with the simple paragraph, 'I was born on _____ in _____, West Virginia, the _____ of _____ children. My parents were _____ and _____, and my grandparents were _____, _____, _____, and _____. My father worked as a _____, and my mother was a _____. I started school at _____ in 19__. My first teacher was _____."

That is not too complicated for anyone, but I dare say there are families out there who don't even know these simple facts about their own parents. This little paragraph was meant to prime the pump, and in one case out of the four, it did just that. Admittedly, I shamed Mom into it. Every time I talked with her, I asked how much she had written. For at least a month, the somewhat snippy response was, "Nothing! I don't know what to write."

After I squeezed the name of her first teacher out of her, I pumped her for more information. It turns out she didn't really remember much about her first teacher, but another later one was her "favorite." He had an injury from World War I but was evidently a kind man and quite a dancer, demonstrating the Charleston for his students at the drop of a hat. His influence extended past the classroom and he worked hard to find jobs for his students in that isolated Appalachian farm community. "And he was good looking," Mom added with a smile.

"Write that down. Just as you told it to me." I made sure the book was on the table right beside her corner of the sofa, so it was always visible and easily reached. That's all it took. "When I think of something, I have to write it down right then, or I will forget it." Well, join the club, Mom. "I couldn't remember the names of the people who lived down the road who we sold milk to, so I called my cousin Leona last night and asked her. We talked for almost an hour."

Did you now? Dad had been gone for several years and Mom lived alone. She now had something to occupy her time in a more mentally stimulating way than watching the 400th rerun of *The Waltons*. It even initiated telephone conversations with extended family members. I am sure they began, "Danny has me doing this stupid thing, so don't blame me, but do you remember where we went that time with Daddy to get the pop and ice cream for the Fourth of July? The ice cream was on dry ice, remember?" I will accept being that fall guy any day. She died recently, but we will treasure what she accomplished, and she was proud of it. The other three ladies? Well, in baseball batting .300 is usually considered pretty good, but I am only at .250.

The reason this section should come last in your *Book of the Still Living* is that, unlike the other sections, it isn't meant to be finished until *you are*. Keep adding pages. You will likely remember additional things to add after a section is complete (probably while taking a shower or lying in bed wishing you could fall asleep) but that is the advantage of a loose-leaf binder. Just write your new memories and clip the page in as an addendum to the story already told.

Since today's seniors are hip and happenin' tech-savvy oldsters, why not just do this whole thing on your computer, making revision simple? If you are comfortable with that go ahead, but remember someone may suddenly and unexpectedly need access to it and it may be password protected. Documents and even photos can be scanned in. But while I would find existence without .docx tedious and frustrating, there is still good reason for your final opus to be a hard copy. Keeping it handy to write in while you are watching television will lead to more quickly-jotted-down memories than logging in to your laptop. Plus, there is something about having and holding the hand-written labor of a deceased loved one. While a book can be stolen or lost, so can computer files (a revelation, I know!). Maybe a dual approach can work for you, with a handwritten work copy that is regularly transcribed into a digital file when you feel like it; run copies, and hole-punch them into the book.

You may even wish to make copies for your family at some point, absent all the passwords and other confidential information. No, today that does not mean an assembly line of people to collate and hole punch. Self-publishing has eliminated the need for all that dreariness. There are many options, but Amazon's Kindle Direct Publishing is probably the biggest, and it doesn't cost a dime until you are ready to buy a single copy, or as many as you need. The process is easy. Convert your file to a .pdf, upload it, create a cover with one of their templates, and your slick paperback will be available in just over a week. For about $5.00 a copy plus postage (with no minimum number to buy!), your personal 100-page *Book of the Still Living* can join Danielle Steel and John Gresham on every bookshelf in the family. Talk about inexpensive Christmas gifts!

You may find other uses for this process. Both sides of my family produced a family cookbook years ago. We all submitted recipes, a cousin typed them all up and ran copies and hole punched all the sheets and assembled them into binders. Over the years, others in the family wanted the cookbook, which meant disassembling it, making more copies, punching, assembling, again and again. When I became familiar with self-publishing technology, I scanned the old pages, wrote an introduction, and combined them with a simple cover filled with family photos. Now, anyone in the family can order a large format copy of *An Appalachian Family Table: The Combined Kuhn and Bennett Families of Southern West Virginia Cookbook* for $12. No more assembly, copying, or punching. Try it with something you have lying around (that is either your own work or not copyrighted, of course).

That fill-in-the-blank paragraph that got Mom started is called a *writing prompt*, and you can make them up yourself. You may want to divide them into timeline sections to make it more organized. Take the 1970s for example. Woo hoo! Now there was a decade. I began it as a chubby pubescent farm boy looking for pop bottles to turn back in for deposit hoping to raise weenie roast money after feeding the hogs and hoeing potatoes, but then ended it as an angsty newly minted college graduate with lots of hair and no girlfriend.

You can go year by year: 1970 writing prompts may include your school and teacher (which most of us can remember) and that may trigger a linear progression of memories. *Sixth grade...that was the year I was in the double classroom with the big folding doors and had that crabby Mrs. Anderson. I remember her reaction when I got ink on Ronnie's shirt, the kid who sat in front of me. My brother got married that year and it was the first time I ever had on a suit. I thought those little Styrofoam bells on the wedding cake were sugar and tried to eat one of them.* And on and on and on. Then there was 1971, and getting thrown into junior high gym class with practically grown men who had failed so many terms they were able to drive to school. *-shudder-*

What I would still like to do

Let's be optimistic. It's the *Book of the Still Living*, so you're not done with everything quite yet. This section pushes you to think about what is important enough to do before the sand runs out. Rank them if you can, tell why they are important to you, and why you haven't already done them. Who would you want to accompany you? What would need to happen to accomplish those things? How can obstacles be overcome? Not only might it inspire you to prioritize and use the time you have left most wisely, but it may also later give your loved ones more insight into what's truly important to *themselves* and lessen regrets about things left undone.

Anyone want to join me in Iceland to see the Aurora Borealis? Or the giant sequoias in California? I have been to both places more than once, but the schedule didn't include seeing those sights. There is no reason to think those things are now out of reach for a nearsighted mid-60s writer guy. But my Disneyland date with

Laurie Partridge is probably now a no-go, since we are both married. Well, Susan Dey and I are, anyhow. Dream big but be realistic.

Now can you see this exercise is as much for you as it is for your left-behinds? It demands more mental calisthenics than watching television and may help keep you sharp. It can give you an added sense of accomplishment and purpose. Even if you think these memories will not be of interest to a single other human being, they are yours and deserve a chance to outlive you. While we should stop being obsessed with trying influence what happens after we die, crafting your own written narrative to be left behind is something totally under your control.

Begin your own *Book of the Still Living* today. If some of us devote even a quarter of the time we spend scrolling Facebook to something that can benefit both us and our family and even someday introduce us to as-of-yet unborn descendants, the personal importance of the work could rival *Angela's Ashes* or *A Movable Feast*. If you haven't read either of those, give up another quarter of your Facebook time and do so.

One last thought about leaving it all behind: is there something, perhaps, you *don't* want to leave? Or at least, be found after you're gone? Think about it right now: if my house, car, storage unit, etc. were completely emptied out by my descendants today, would there be things I would not want them to see? As research heavy as this book is, I can't give you an estimate of how many of us to whom that might apply.

Er…I use "us" there in the universal sense, of course.

There may be parts of our personal lives we want to *keep personal* and confidential from our closest kin, even in death. There are many stories about spouses or children finding things that disturbed them in a deceased loved one's personal effects, and most probably go untold through embarrassment. As you can guess, many of those things involve sex. Sex toys, fetish gear, pornography, photos or film of the decedent with a lover could all be lurking out there in closets, attics, and garage lockers (not yours or mine, of course, but speaking theoretically). Pulling back the clothes in Pawpaw's closet to load them up for Goodwill and finding a life-sized silicone sex doll named Jordan (according to the tag on the nape of his/her neck) with interchangeable male/female groin bits hiding in the back could be a shocker. Does Goodwill even take those? And what about his stash of medicinal weed in a backward state where it's illegal?

Then there are less interesting things that are still problematic, such as stolen property that has been hidden for decades or illegal firearms.

I had never seen it before, and it looked old. It was in the bottom of Dad's wooden tool chest and I have no idea if it worked, but it seemed like it would. How on earth did he come by a sawed-off shotgun with the serial number filed off? I knew it could cause trouble, so I called the city cops. They came and took it and thanked me. I made sure to get a receipt for it. Now, chances are probably good it ended up in one of their tool chests as a conversation piece, but at least it isn't going to cause me any headache. -Male

There are also many stories about things people are happy to find, like envelopes of money. I live in an area subject to hurricanes, and I keep some cash on hand in case card readers are down or other events make credit cards temporarily useless. We all feel we can outsmart a burglar by hiding valuable things around the house. But think: if I were not here an hour from now, would there be things I want to leave behind that might go unfound? Should those gold coins behind the mudroom baseboard really stay there until the next owners of the house remodel it? There are probably millions of dollars that have gone to landfills over the years in false-bottomed drawers, behind pictures of dogs playing poker, and the linings of drapes that were quite stylish in 1975. Valuable things do your loved ones no good in the dumpster or on the Goodwill shelf. If something is well hidden, you are at risk of forgetting about it or losing it yourself as your memory fades. Do something about it now.

As to the embarrassing things, it's comforting to think you will have time just before dying to get rid of them. It's also a foolish risk. Maybe give your descendants credit that they know you are human. And heck, Jordan cost $3,000. Your great-grandchildren might fight over him/her (as a Halloween decoration, of course).

This chapter has been a difficult journey for me and perhaps parts of it was uncomfortable for you as well, I suspect. It has probably caused us both to relive some tough moments and think harder about our own mortality than we like. I have difficulty writing anything without seasoning it with at least a dash of humor and irony, so I hope you haven't found anything to be disrespectful. Death is one of the things we all have in common, no matter how rich or poor, popular or isolated, healthy or sickly, sophisticated or common, beautiful or homely, loved or reviled we may be. In the end, it is, quite literally, the one thing that brings us all together. Thank you for sticking with me. I'll see you on the other side. Maybe.

THE TAKEAWAY

You are planning to die, but are you *planning* to die? There are a thousand different scenarios of how we will breathe our last and what happens then, and you can't anticipate them all. Having as many contingencies covered as you can is good for your family, but it is even better for yourself.

Do what you can, and then try to let it go. We aren't used to not being able to control things if we just work hard enough, spend enough money, do enough research, and enlist enough help. That was Middle Life, and most of us eventually move on from that. We all depended on others for care and love when we were babies, and we may do so again by necessity in Old Life.

Don't neglect telling your story. Leaving it for someone else is optional, but you have thoughts, memories, and wisdom that should be passed on. It's easy to do so, and helps you come to terms with your life in the process, even if no one else ever sees it. *The Book of the Still Living* is more for yourself than anyone else. The dedicated notebook is important because it can become your companion, your special project. Resolve to begin it today or tomorrow, no excuses.

Don't beat yourself up over having fear, anxiety, and sadness over knowing death is closer than ever before. We all do, even if we don't admit it. But also don't be reluctant to seek professional help if it begins to impact your enjoyment of today. Allow it to motivate you to do the things you want to do while you still have time.

My final wish for you is that you can do them with someone you love.

Note concerning italicized quotes: While some are directly from writings, personal conversations, or social media, others are composites enhanced by the author to illustrate a point. All come from true expression, but may have been rearranged, recombined, or reconfigured.

IF YOU FOUND THIS WORK HELPFUL: Since we no longer talk with one another about books anymore, please do you, me, and your friends a favor by leaving a review of it on Amazon or other review platforms. I sincerely thank you.

Danny Kuhn

COMING SOON FROM THIS AUTHOR: ***The Book of the Still Living.*** **We are all planning to die, but are we** ***planning*** **to die? This large-format manual helps you plan and organize all the important information your "left behinds" will need to know, plus things about yourself to leave as a legacy. It also helps you devise a strategy for keeping usernames, passwords, account numbers, and other "where did I put that?" information accessible when needed, all in one handy place. It will become the** ***Book of You.*** **Watch for it from Favoritetrainers.com Books!**

REFERENCE LIST

CHAPTER 1

1. University of Michigan's *Institute for Healthcare Policy and Innovation's National Poll on Healthy Aging*
2. A Study of Sexuality and Health among Older Adults in the United States [*New England Journal of Medicine.* 2007; 357: 662-774 by S. Lindau, L. Schumm, E. Laumann, W. Levinson, C. O'Muircheartaigh, and L. Waite)
3. *The Journals of Gerontology, Series B: Psychological and Social Sciences*, June 22, 2017
4. Allen MS. Sexual Activity and Cognitive Decline in Older Adults. *Arch Sex Behav.* 2018 Aug;47(6):1711-1719. doi: 10.1007/s10508-018-1193-8. Epub 2018 May 16. PMID: 29767822.
5. W. Padoani, M. Dello Buona, and P. Marietta et al., Influence of Cognitive Status on the Sexual Life of 352 Elderly Italians Aged 65-105 Years (published in *Gerontology*, 2000
6. Smith L, Yang L, Veronese N, Soysal P, Stubbs B, and Jackson SE in *Sex Med.* (2019 Mar;7(1):11-18. doi: 10.1016/j.esxm.2018.11.001. Epub 2018 Dec 13. PMID: 30554952; PMCID: PMC6377384).
7. (Julie Frappier, Isabelle Toupin, Joseph J. Levy, Mylene Aubertin-Leheudre, and Antony D. Karelis, published in the journal *PLOS ONE* 10-24-2013)
8. Pallesen S, Waage S, Thun E, Andreassen CS, Bjorvatn B. A national survey on how sexual activity is perceived to be associated with sleep. Sleep and Biological Rhythms. 2020;18(1):65–72)
9. Ramadhan MA, Hashim HT. The Effects of Sexual Frequency and Immune Boosting Mineral Intake on Immune Status in COVID-19 Susceptible Individuals. *Fertil Steril.* 2021 Sep;116(3):e113. doi: 10.1016/j.fertnstert.2021.07.316. Epub 2021 Sep 17. PMCID: PMC8446874)
10. Kanter G, Rogers RG, Pauls RN, Kammerer-Doak D, Thakar R. A strong pelvic floor is associated with higher rates of sexual activity in women with pelvic floor disorders. *Int Urogynecol J.* 2015 Jul;26(7):991-6. doi: 10.1007/s00192-014-2583-7. Epub 2015 May 21. PMID: 25994625; PMCID: PMC4573594
11. Rider JR, Wilson KM, Sinnott JA, Kelly RS, Mucci LA, Giovannucci EL. Ejaculation Frequency and Risk of Prostate

Cancer: Updated Results with an Additional Decade of Follow-up. *Eur Urol.* 2016 Dec;70(6):974-982. Doi 10.1016/j. eururo.2016.03.027. Epub 2016 Mar 28. PMID: 27033442; PMCID: PMC5040619)

12. Pornography Consumption in People of Different Age Groups: An Analysis Based on Gender, Contents, and Consequences (Ballester-Arnal, Garcia-Barba, Castro-Calvo, Gimenez-Garcia and Gil-Llario, *Sexuality Research and Social Policy,* May 2022

13. Aleksandra Dwulit and Piotr Rzymski published as The Potential Associations of Pornography Use with Sexual Dysfunctions: An Integrative Literature Review of Observational Studies in *The Journal of Clinical Medicine*, 2019

14. Kohut and Fisher, *The impact of brief exposure to sexually explicit video clips on partnered female clitoral self-stimulation, orgasm, and sexual satisfaction.* Department of Psychology, Western University, London Ontario, got rather specific with their Volume 22 (Spring 2013) article in *The Canadian Journal of Human Sexuality:*

15. Click Bait: Problematic Internet Pornography Use Among Older Adults (Tao, Moreno, and Morgan, *The American Journal of Geriatric Psychology*, March 2019:

16. Is Internet Pornography Causing Sexual Dysfunction? A Review with Clinical Reports (Park BY, Wilson G, Berger J, Christman M, Reina B, Bishop F, Klam WP, Doan AP. *Behav Sci (Basel).* 2016 Aug 5;6(3):17. doi: 10.3390/bs6030017. Erratum in: *Behav Sci (Basel).* 2018 Jun 01;8(6): PMID: 27527226; PMCID: PMC5039517)

17. EO Laumann and LJ Waite (Laumann EO, Waite LJ. Sexual dysfunction among older adults: prevalence and risk factors from a nationally representative U.S. probability sample of men and women 57-85 years of age. *Journal of Sex Med.* 2008 Oct;5(10):2300-11. doi: 10.1111/j.1743-6109.2008.00974.x. Epub 2008 Aug 12. PMID: 18702640; PMCID: PMC2756968).

18. *Lovehoney* reported in *The Mirror* (Shivali Best, April 17, 2019)

19. Use and Procurement of Additional Lubricants for Male and Female Condoms, WHO/UNFPA/FHI360, *World Health Organization*, 2012.

20. Smith, Bergeron, Goltz, Coffey, and Boolani (Smith ML, Bergeron CD, Goltz HH, Coffey T, Boolani A. Sexually Transmitted Infection Knowledge among Older Adults:

Psychometrics and Test-Retest Reliability. *Int J Environ Res Public Health.* 2020 Apr 3;17(7):2462. doi: 10.3390/ijerph17072462. PMID: 32260298; PMCID: PMC7177870)

21. *IJIR: Your Sexual Medicine Journal*, March 2020
22. David Frederick, Janet Lever, Brian Gillespie, and Justin Garcia, What Keeps Passion Alive? Sexual Satisfaction Is Associated With Sexual Communication, Mood Setting, Sexual Variety, Oral Sex, Orgasm, and Sex Frequency in a National U. S. Study published in *The Journal of Sex Research* Vol. 54 (2017)

CHAPTER 3

23. C. C. Tangney (*Cardiovascular benefits and risks of moderate alcohol consumption*) and K. J. Mukamal (*Overview of the risks and benefits of alcohol consumption*), referenced by The May Clinic
24. Harvard Medical School (*Staying Healthy: 11 Ways to Curb Your Drinking,* May 2022)
25. (Gruber SA, Sagar KA, Dahlgren MK, Gonenc A, Smith RT, Lambros AM, Cabrera KB, Lukas SE. The Grass Might Be Greener: Medical Marijuana Patients Exhibit Altered Brain Activity and Improved Executive Function after 3 Months of Treatment. *Front Pharmacol.* 2018 Jan 17;8:983. doi: 10.3389/fphar.2017.00983. PMID: 29387010; PMCID: PMC5776082.
26. Results from the 2018 National Survey on Drug Use and Health (Rockville, MD: *Center for Behavioral Health Statistics and Quality, Substance Abuse and Mental Health Services Administration*).
27. Why were millions of opioid pills sent to a West Virginia town of 3,000? By Chris McGreal in *The Guardian*, October 2, 2019
28. Culberson, J. W. and Ziska, M. Prescription drug misuses/abuse in the elderly, *Geriatrics*, 2008.

CHAPTER 4

29. T. Hull and J. M. Church, Colonoscopy—How difficult, how painful? *Cleveland Clinic Foundation*, 1994

30. E. Samami, Z. Shahhosseini, and E. Forouzan, The Effects of Psychological Interventions on Menopausal Hot Flashes: A Systematic Review, *National Library of Medicine,* May 2022.
31. If Pneumonia is the 'Old Man's Friend,' Should it be Prevented by Vaccination? An Ethical Analysis, by Richard Kent Zimmerman (*NIH National Library of Medicine, National Center for Biotechnology Information*, March 23, 2005).
32. Drs. Karina De Sousa, Vinaya Manchaiah, David Moore, et al *Journal of the American Medical Association (JAMA) Otolaryngology, Head and Neck Surgery,* April 2023
33. *Harmonized Cognitive Assessment Protocol Project*, University of Michigan, 2017

CHAPTER 5

34. Ariella, Sky. The 10 Largest Nursing Home Companies in the United States. *Zippia*, April 2023

CHAPTER 6

35. National Academies of Sciences, Engineering, and Medicine, *Social Isolation and Loneliness in Older Adults: Opportunities for the Health Care System* (2020)
36. *Growing Young: How Friendship, Optimism, and Kindness Can Help You Live to 100* (Penguin Random House Canada, 2020).

CHAPTER 7

37. Ware, Bronnie. *The Top Five Regrets of the Dying: A Life Transformed by the Dearly Departing* (Hay House, August 2019
38. Pink, Daniel H. *The Power of Regret: How Looking Backward Moves Us Forward* (Riverhead Books, February 2022
39. Raichien, David; Klimentidis, Yann, Sayer, M. Katherine, and Alexander, Gene, "Leisure-time sedentary behaviors are differentially associated with all-cause dementia regardless of engagement in physical activity *Proceedings of the National Academy of Sciences*

CHAPTER 8

40. Hashemi A, Oroojan AA, Rassouli M, Ashrafizadeh H. Explanation of near-death experiences: a systematic analysis of case reports and qualitative research. *Front Psychol.* 2023 Apr 20;14:1048929. doi: 10.3389/fpsyg.2023.1048929. PMID: 37151318; PMCID: PMC10158795.
41. Parnia S, Spearpoint K, Gabriele de Vos G, Fenwick P, Goldberg, D, Yang J, Zhu, et al. AWARE-Awareness during Resuscitation-A prospective study. *Resuscitation,* Vol 85, Issue 12 December 2014 pp 1799-1805
42. Sade RM. Brain death, cardiac death, and the dead donor rule. *J S C Med Assoc.* 2011 Aug;107(4):146-9. PMID: 22057747; PMCID: PMC3372912
43. Yadav, K., Gabler, N., Cooney, E. et al, Approximately One in Three US Adults Completes Any Type of Advance Directive for End-of-Life Care, *Health Affairs*, Vol. 36, No. 7, July 2017

ABOUT THE AUTHOR

Danny Kuhn holds degrees from Marshall and West Virginia Universities. A former social worker, high school science teacher, and Federal Probation Officer, he now writes in Myrtle Beach, South Carolina. His second novel, *Thoreau's Wound: A Novel of Ireland and America*, was published by Knox Robinson Publishing, London and Atlanta, in 2017 with a foreword by Alphie McCourt (brother of Angela's Ashes' Frank McCourt). His *Daily Inspiration for Progressive America* offers page-a-day reading with uplifting history, quotes, and analysis. *Fezziwig: A Life* (Knox Robinson Publishing, London and Atlanta) is his first novel. It gives a full life to one of Dickens's most beloved minor characters, and has been reviewed by James Burke, Adam Hart-Davis, Nick Barratt, and Anton Gill. Danny is also the author of *Fresh History Brewed Daily: Raleigh County (WV) People, Places, Happenings* (Favoritetrainers.com Books, 2015), *O, Mountaineers! Noted (or Notorious) West Virginians* (and *Volume II, African American West Virginians*) and contributor and co-editor of *Mountain Mysts: Myth and Fantasy of the Mountains* (Headline Books, 2015), *Not Taking a Fence - Verses, Stories, and Memories from the Heart of Appalachia* (Favoritetrainers.com Books, 2015), and *Writing for Clarity* (Favoritetrainers.com Books, 2017). His *Tales Irish* (Favoritetrainers.com Books, 2017) is an international collection in collaboration with 20 Irish authors, and offers haunting tales of Ireland, past and present. *Not a Dog Person,* released in 2023 (Favoritetrainers.com Books, is his latest work. His articles have appeared in *Commonweal* and *The Sun.*

ABOUT THE ILLUSTRATIONS

Almost everyone agrees, it seems, that Mark Twain was America's greatest humorist. If asked, I preface his name by saying "greatest *19th Century* humorist" because of James Grover Thurber, who died in November 1961, back when I was a toddler.

Yes, Twain made me think more. But, since I discovered him when I was in junior high school, Thurber has made me laugh much, much more than Twain. His stories gave us, in large part, the kind of modern, witty, urbane, ironic humor that is today's standard, yet I feel he is underappreciated, understudied, and underread.

If you are reading these words and have not read the marvelous short story collections by James Thurber, nor his cartoon collections, please do so. Your life will be fuller for it.

In the early 1990s, my family and I visited relatives in Columbus, Ohio, and top on my sightseeing list was to visit Thurber's birthplace, 251 Parsons Avenue. On a hot and humid August day, we loaded the girls into the Plymouth Voyager and set off with a city roadmap, in those pre-GPS days. It wasn't hard to find…the overgrown vacant lot beside Interstate 71. No marker, no monument, no anything.

I knew I was missing something. Consulting the phonebook (trees used to give their lives for those), I found the Thurber Club and called, hoping to contact fellow devotees. A gentleman answered "Turber Club. Can I help you?" I heard a juke box and the *click* of pool balls in the background. Strike two.

Finally, I found the Thurber House, beautifully restored at 77 Jefferson Avenue. James's family moved into the brick home while he was a student at *the* Ohio State University. And yes, this was the house the ghost once got into to terrorize his family. And it satisfied my Thurberish longings, being a museum and literary center, both showcasing Thurber's life and work as well as supporting other aspiring writers. Visit it if you can.

While I have proclaimed Thurber to be the Father of Modern American Humor, my tribute to him in telling my true story involves what is sometimes considered his lesser literary contribution: his cartoons. Their popularity during the 1930s-50s surprised even him, since he was not, shall we say, and extremely talented or gifted artist. Some, it can objectively be said, look like scrawls. It is possible we would never even have seen them had not his friend E. B. White (*Charlotte's Web*) plucked some of James's doodles out of the trash at The New Yorker and submitted them for publication. His lack of formal art training was exacerbated by his being plagued by poor eyesight, stemming from playing William Tell with his brother when James was seven years old. In later years, he was effectively blind.

I almost never read a book twice, with Dickens and Thurber being exceptions. So many books, so little time, you know? But his cartoons are old friends to whom I return again and again.

Thurber found great humor in the indignities of aging. Most are my paltry and juvenile re-workings of his unnamed characters and locations to fit my story, (including the couple in bed, though the seal barking has been replaced by the hmmmm of a vibrator) but, trust me, it is done with all honor, respect, and love for James Thurber and his work. It is, to the last word and scrawl, brilliant. He was a genius. Given the subject, I think he would approve. If not, his ghost may get in and let me know and, perhaps, in the afterlife, I can make him a heavenly gin and tonic to compensate.

Cover designer SETH ELLISON is a graduate of the Savannah College of Art and Design and The University of the Arts, Philadelphia. You can view his artwork at www.sethellison.com.

www.ingramcontent.com/pod-product-compliance
Lightning Source LLC
Chambersburg PA
CBHW062051270326
41931CB00013B/3034